Praise for *Find Your Food Voice*

"*Find Your Food Voice* by Julie Duffy Dillon is a compassionate and empowering guide for anyone struggling with their relationship with food. With her non-diet approach, Julie encourages readers to reconnect with their body's innate wisdom and break free from the harmful cycle of dieting. Through heartfelt letters and real-life stories, this book offers tools for healing and prioritizing body autonomy, making it an invaluable resource for those seeking a more peaceful and joyful connection with food."

Sam Abbott, MSEd, RD, LDN, Registered Dietitian Nutritionist

"Julie Duffy Dillon believes you! She believes every one of your words that describe the painful experiences that have kept you trapped in shame and suffering throughout your dieting life. With an engaging and readable manner, *Find Your Food Voice* will guide you back to your eating wisdom that has been confiscated by diet culture. Written with deep honesty and compassion, this book will challenge you to confront the lies that you've been fed by the diet and wellness industries. With renewed trust in your inner voice, you will build a joyful relationship with food, that embraces you with the safety and freedom that you've been missing."

Elyse Resch, MS, RDN, CEDS-C, Co-author and creator of Intuitive Eating

Find Your Food Voice

Find Your Food Voice

JULIE DUFFY DILLON

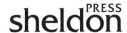
sheldon PRESS

First published by Sheldon Press in 2025
An imprint of John Murray Press

1

Copyright © Julie Duffy Dillon 2025

This book is for information or educational purposes only and is not intended to act
as a substitute for medical advice or treatment. Any person with a condition requiring
medical attention should consult a qualified medical practitioner or suitable therapist.

A CIP catalogue record for this title is available from the British Library

Library of Congress Control Number: 2024950095
Trade Paperback ISBN 978 1 399 81365 5
ebook ISBN 978 1 399 81366 2

Typeset by KnowledgeWorks Global Ltd.

Printed and bound in the United States of America

John Murray Press policy is to use papers that are natural, renewable and recyclable
products and made from wood grown in sustainable forests. The logging and
manufacturing processes are expected to conform to the environmental
regulations of the country of origin.

John Murray Press
Carmelite House
50 Victoria Embankment
London EC4Y 0DZ

123 S. Broad St., Ste 2750
Philadelphia, PA 19109

The authorised representative in the EEA is Hachette Ireland, 8 Castlecourt Centre,
Dublin 15, D15 XTP3, Ireland (email: info@hbgi.ie)

www.sheldonpress.co.uk

John Murray Press, part of Hodder & Stoughton Limited
An Hachette UK company

For Corrina and Oliver

Acknowledgments

I have wanted to write a book since my sixth-grade teacher, Miss Mosconi, had me read aloud (while I was probably in full-on panic attack mode and blushing in embarrassment) an essay about a rooster sitting on a pile of eggs. In the essay, in my shaky 12-year-old voice, I explored feminism and men doing the heavy lifting of breaking apart the patriarchy. Miss Mosconi pulled me aside later and said she wanted to read my book someday. I still remember how she looked me in the eye and said, "I mean it." Thank you, Miss Mosconi, for believing in me even then. Thank you, Rachel Landes from Sheldon Press and the entire Sheldon team, for taking a risk on me and helping me make writing a book a reality for me.

My heart fills with gratitude as I think about every person supporting me as I wrote this book. My constant cheerleaders have been my children. Corrina, you are my biggest fan and I love you so much. Thank you for encouraging me even when times are tough. Please know you teach me more than you'll ever know just by being you. I am grateful you are you. Oliver, you have helped me better understand how to notice, name, and accept feelings even when they clash. You are better at feeling than most adults; this is your strength. I love you. I am so grateful you are you.

To my parents and my brothers and their families, thank you for supporting me and cheering me on. Thank you to my children's father, Kevin Dillon, for always supporting my work and encouraging me to write this book. Thank you to my girls—Kelly Kocher, Anne Smith, Katie McCrone, Lori Brecht, and Julie Brown—our text thread always makes me laugh until I cry. I love you.

In January 2020, I joined a neighborhood book club. I was yearning for new friends and laughter, even though I wasn't the biggest reader. We all know what happened over the next few months, and this book club became my survival alliance. Tammy Shaney-Grubbs, Lauren Shaney-Grubbs, Stephanie Held, Jen Nixon, Jennifer Rogers, Kate Guthrie, Brandon Fox, Anna Martinek-Jenne, and Allison Walker—thank you for being my dependable do-or-die friends. Thank you for teaching me community and that I am worthy of support. You were the first people

I told about this book and your cheers kept me going. I know I am never alone because you are just a text away.

Around Chapter 5, you may notice a subtle flair enter my writing because that is when I met Jorge Gutiérrez-Marmolejo. Thank you, my love, for being my loudest listener. Your kindness and conversations helped me get through every step of this. Our time together has made this book much more *me*, and I look forward to sharing countless meals and *sobremesas* with you.

I couldn't have written this book without the support from my work colleagues who are also dear friends. I leave you a desperate Voxer message or lengthy text and you always know how to help me pick up the pieces and get back moving forward with compassion. Lindsay Stenovec, Jennifer McGurk, and Sumner Brooks—thank you for listening to my too long Voxers and helping me visualize the Voice Finder Cord and so many other important aspects of *Find Your Food Voice*. Christie Hunter—you're my dietitian cheerleader and always there to lift me up when I am down. Thank you for being such a great friend. To my local non-diet colleagues—Megan Hadley, Laura Watson, Deb Benfield, Jessie Spence, Donetta Floyd, Heather Kitchen, April Forsbrey, and Brett Debney—thank you for all the conversations and encouragement over the years. Thank you, Kimmie Singh, for striking up a conversation at UNCG after class. I have learned much from you since then, and you have made the nutrition and non-diet space better, safer, and more inclusive.

Thank you, Beth Rosen, my HAES bestie, for being a supportive and patient listener in work and life. Thank you, Laura Burns, for trusting me to help you build a PCOS support community. I miss our craft hangouts and conversations!

Thank you to all the dietitian podcasters, content creators, and conference connectors who have taught me and made me laugh. I live for the opportunities to chat with you in person over a meal. Marci Evans, Fiona Sutherland, Christy Harrison, Christyna Johnson, Nancy Clark, Dawn Clifford, Jessica Setnick, Glenys Oyston, Aaron Flores and so many others—let's do this soon! Thank you, Elyse Resch and Evelyn Tribole, for writing the *Intuitive Eating* book—your work saved me from quitting dietetics, and I have always felt supported by you as I make my way into non-diet work.

At my first Binge Eating Disorder Conference in the early 2000s, I met Marilyn Wann and Deb Burgard. From their suggestion, I started to learn more about body liberation from fat activists, many of whom held multiple identities where naming diet industry harms put them in harm's way. Without the heroic work of Black queer body liberation activists in the 1960s, I wouldn't have been rescued from diet harm and learned how to help people navigate *I-Should-Eat* recovery. I appreciate I will never know the names of many of the people who helped me write this book and I am grateful for their continued impact on my life. A big thank-you to present-day body liberation activists who have impacted my life and helped me write this book. Thank you in particular to Ragen Chastain, SJ Belmonte, Jessica Wilson, Lindley Ashline, Bri Campos, Da'Shaun L. Harrison, Elizabeth Armstrong, Marilyn Wann, Sabrina Strings, Roxanne Gay, Alishia McCullough, Dani Adriana, Jes Baker, and many others—your work has impacted my life and work. Thank you for putting yourself out there and taking the risk. If you are reading this and don't know one or more of these folks, buy their books, support their Patreon, and pay them to learn more about how to help fellow Voice Finders access life without another *I-Should-Eat* script!

Getting through writing a book is its own full-time job—on top of another one! I couldn't have gotten through this without the support of Rachel Popik, Coleen Bremner, Yeli Cruz, and Tabitha Andrews—people who have worked behind the scenes in my business over the past few years. I am a mess constantly and grateful they have helped me get out of my own way to get things turned in on time.

Thank you to my supervisors over the years—all who have guided me while I bawled my eyes out. Thank you, Deb Benfield, Deb Burgard, Lisa Pearl, Tammy Beasley, Linda Makinson, Ann White, Shawn Spurgeon, and many others for leading me and helping me to trust my process. Thank you to any colleague or client who has given me feedback. Thank you for believing in me enough to tell me the things I needed to hear. You have helped me grow to be a kinder human.

Thank you to those who have let me supervise them. What a privilege watching you become the clinician the world needs.

I would never recommend writing a book without individual psychotherapy. Thank you to all my therapists, especially Helen

Campbell, who have helped me heal my voice. I couldn't have written a word without your belief in me. Thank you for showing me how brave I can be.

Lastly, thank you to all of you who have sat on my green office couch as a client. You were a part of this book, and you floated through my mind as I typed. I could not have done any of this if you didn't trust me with your vulnerabilities. It was a privilege to hold space with you and witness your process to finding your Food Voice. When we pass each other in the grocery store or in a restaurant, know I am rooting for you. Even though we probably don't speak in these moments, I am proud of you. You are still very brave.

Contents

Prologue

Voice Finders

Throughout this book I have drawn upon the voices, lived experiences, and wisdom from 25 years of clinical practice. Here I introduce you to these courageous Voice Finders, together with the first Dear Food letter they wrote. Please note each client described here is not based on any one person and purely fictional.

Matilda

Pronouns: she/her

Identities: 20-year-old college student at a prestigious private university. She was adopted at birth and, unaware of ethnic identity, raised by white parents. She has recently been diagnosed with polycystic ovary syndrome (PCOS) and has identified as plus size since middle school.

> Dear Food,
>
> I have tried cutting out carbs, sugar, pasta, and anything white flour–based for years and my weight is still going up. When I ask doctors for a solution, I can tell on their face they don't believe how little I eat. Should I look into surgery? I don't think I can cut any more foods out or exercise more. I feel stuck and alone.
>
> Love,
> Matilda

Rae

Pronouns: they/them

Identities: 43-year-old white, trans-masculine, nonbinary accountant with PCOS. They identify as superfat.

Dear Food,

   We have had a long twisted road together, and I can't remember a time when I wasn't stressing myself out about how much to eat. Even as a kid, food was a fight. Will I ever enjoy eating?

   Yours truly,
   Rae

Paul

Pronouns: he/him
   Identities: 37-year-old cisgender, heterosexual lawyer married to Gene (she/they). Paul identifies as neurodivergent and as a food addict.

Dear Food,

   I fucking hate you. I know I have to be with you sometimes, yet it is always a struggle. I can't trust myself around you and can only manage my job if you are behind lock and key. Literally.

   Best,
   Paul

Elena

Pronouns: she/her
   Identities: 24-year-old cisgender new teacher. She identifies as Mexican-American and her parents immigrated to the United States from Mexico before she was born. She lives with pre-diabetes.

Dear Food,

   I am a mess. I have worked so hard to get through school only now to be a failure with my weight gain and diabetes diagnosis. My parents have lived with it, too, and they are constantly nagging me to cut out more foods. Food feels pointless but I feel like it can be more.

   Sincerely,
   Elena

Keisha

Pronouns: she/her

Identities: 53-year-old Black technology company executive. She identifies as fat and is mom to Traci.

> Dear Food,
>
> I see how little Traci eats and worry it is because of me. Well, not really me, but how the world sees me. I desperately want to find a way to help her not starve herself and be safe. Is there a way?
>
> Love,
> Keisha

Traci

Pronouns: she/her

Identities: 15-year-old mixed-race high-school student recently diagnosed with anorexia nervosa.

> Dear Food,
>
> What's the point of you? You will just make me overweight like my mom, and I see how the world treats her. My mom worries about me, yet I want her to understand I will do everything I can to eat less and less of food until I am no longer able to be harmed.
>
> XOXO,
> Traci

1

Start Here

Dear Food,

When I was a new mom struggling with sleep-deprivation and thoughts of inadequacy, I got a chance to travel to Europe with a friend. I hadn't had a moment to myself in 18 months, and then I flew to Paris. Paris felt like the opposite of my then current reality: a romantic, eclectic, energizing, *adult* place. I didn't have to change a diaper, and no screaming baby needed me. The sights, smells, and sounds all fed me.

Food, high five for that amazing banana-and-Nutella crepe when I got lost in Paris's Latin Quarter.

Do you remember how I was crying? Not because of my constant feelings of failure that came with motherhood. This time I was so happy! So happy to be lost and alone, and no one could find me. I was so grateful for the *moment* and myself. I was literally blissful being *me*, and strangely, eating such a lovely iconic item of French street food helped deliver that experience.

We haven't been properly introduced, Food. My name is Julie, and I'm a registered dietitian.

Thank you for avocados, olives, and French fries. Thank you for energizing me with calories after I gave birth, which, let me tell you, felt like a marathon. Do you remember the giggles my husband and I had while we took our first bites of wedding cake? Who was the first to smash it into whose face? Or the soothing texture and temperature of tomato soup with grilled cheese as our marriage ended? I have continued to be thankful to this day for the leftover spaghetti and meatballs I ate early in the morning after learning the 2016 US presidential election results. As I cried for all who would be impacted, that warm emotional eating got me through that moment.

Food, you have brought me a connection to joy. You're a vessel to experiencing life in its most important and mundane moments. You soothe in just one bite.

You may be wondering why I'm writing … so here it goes. I have studied food and eating behavior for over 20 years. I am fascinated with how and why we eat and the emotional complexity of our individual and collective relationship with food.

Ellyn Satter says: "When we take the joy out of eating, nutrition suffers."

And we are suffering, Food.

Have you heard about all these diets? *All* the diets? We have keto, low-calorie, low-fat, low-carb, paleo, and intermittent fasting. We also have this weird one called "clean eating." So, if I'm not clean eating, does that mean I'm dirty? We have hidden ones, like "lifestyle change" and "just eating healthily." Or injections of medications designed for diabetes yet used as an instrument for thin compliance.

I believe these ideas start out being about health, but things are getting bad … *really* bad.

The first few years I was a dietitian, I worked with adults trying to lose weight. I also worked with higher-weight kids. I saw people trying desperately to lose weight in any way possible. I also saw them beat themselves up, only to witness healthcare providers pushing them when they were down.

Literally, higher-weight people are given less care and treated differently.

For a long time, I was sucked into this way of thinking, too. We pushed folks to try harder, persuaded them that dieting would make them healthier. When people, some of them children, got weighed in, and we saw they had gained weight, our eyes communicated our disappointment. Many never came back. I never understood why.

I feel much shame today, knowing what I know now.

Eventually, I started to notice the mind-fuck that dieting brings to the participant. It's a seductive fantasy initially… the first days are good and feel like a success. Dieters hear encouraging words and, as they start to lose weight, they describe feeling seen for the first time. As the diet—and it never matters which one—continues, just about everyone hits a roadblock. Maybe a week in, or six months, or a year, yet eventually, they all hit something that makes all the weight come back, plus more.

Food, I thought I was going crazy. Then I did some research and looked into the statistics. Three to 5 percent of dieters keep the weight off two to five years post-diet. This was the first time I realized it wasn't me; it wasn't my clients; and it wasn't your fault either, Food.

Who or what was to blame? Diets.

Food, you'd be proud of me. I don't teach diets anymore, and I'm teaching other healthcare providers to do the same. I have found other fat-positive practitioners, and they've supported and supervised me to help people heal their relationship with you!

I know it sounds weird to think of a relationship with food, but there are many reasons to do this. First, we make over 200 eating decisions a day. We think about you *a lot*. Second, I have found that the way that we experience food mirrors how we relate to others and ourselves. Having a safe and stable way of eating that includes pleasure and promotes health helps us in every other area of life. This may not at first seem to make much sense, yet I hope, over time, it will.

Here's the main reason I'm writing, Food: I'm worried about us. Everyone is so fatphobic and diet-obsessed that we've disconnected from ourselves. Higher-weight people are more than just teased for their body size; they are blocked from accessing dignified healthcare and quality of life. Disordered eating is now considered normal eating. More are sick *and* feeling ashamed from all of the rigid food rules. People literally blame themselves for these diet failures when it's really the diet's fault all along.

I think you can help us out, Food. I want people to be able to write *you* a letter detailing what makes eating so tough. I would appreciate it if you could get back to us on some solutions: how to help us get back to enjoying food; how to reconnect us to our own innate wisdom regarding our health. Most importantly, we need

3

help prioritizing healing and a renewed sense of body autonomy. I speak for my fellow humans—we are out of touch with our most precious and innate knowing: our Food Voice.

Warmly,
A concerned dietitian

When I started to see diet's harm

When my boss knocked on my office door, I was expecting her to be disappointed and angry, but I was not expecting to cry. Unfortunately, it was not one of those easy-to-cover-up cries with a tear just rolling gently down my face.

No, this cry was a sob. This was a snotty, out-of-breath cry. One that I had held inside of me for years and held so much shame. I was not expecting to cry, and I was not expecting to make one of the biggest decisions of my life.

I could give you sentence after sentence as to *why* I am against diets and the pursuit of weight loss. I could examine the abundant critical research on the harm of diets and how they promote high blood pressure, high cholesterol, high insulin levels, high blood sugar, and depression. I could go into how diets predict weight gain. Even if I did go through all of this, I appreciate that you, the reader, might still think I was putting my head in the sand or turning a blind eye to the obesity research. Along those same lines, you might also begin to wonder whether I believed the world was flat!

I appreciate a registered dietitian taking a non-diet approach may appear bizarre. From the outside looking in, non-diet nutrition can look a lot like someone who is ignoring research or doesn't think it's important.

Please know that *Find Your Food Voice* is not about ignoring research but rather using it.

As you are holding this book reading its words, I am assuming a few things: Your relationship with food is complicated. You have tried many different ways to eat less but something keeps you from succeeding. When you start a diet, your weight may go down at first, yet every diet seems to come to the same troubling conclusions, such as obsessing over every bite, feelings of shame that follow every *should* that doesn't fix it, and hating your body that won't adhere to the diets everyone else seems to get right.

While I don't think you owe me or anyone the pursuit of health, we can agree on some level we got tangled up with diets because we are seeking health. We want to live longer, and we are told eating properly will help us extend our life. That's why I became a dietitian: I wanted to help clients reach their goals, to thrive, and know that I was rooting for them along the way.

Listening to food experiences showed me the dangers of dieting

One of my favorite parts of being a dietitian is getting to know people. I remember getting in trouble during my dietitian training years because I was spending too much time sitting and talking with patients.

I loved listening to a patient's rich lived experience. I could walk into a hospital room or a training room or clinic or office, and just sit and let someone know I was listening. I seemed to be able to provide space to let people explore, to open up and be real.

I found early on in my career that I felt at home working with people in the throes of the eating disorder continuum. It's something that I found fascinating and which I really enjoyed learning more about. But I didn't always feel that way. Instead, early on I specialized in working with higher-weight kids and their families.

In those years, while working with kids and their families, I noticed that they were not getting compassionate, comprehensive care. I noticed, too, that thin people who had anorexia and bulimia got a lot of sympathy from the medical community while higher-weight clients did not. When reporting on the types of bullying they'd been subjected to, higher-weight kids said they were encouraged to diet, lose weight, and exercise more to prevent the harassment. I witnessed higher-weight people treated like dirt everywhere even in the healthcare setting.

As I listened to the diverse lived experiences coming from higher-weight kids, I picked up on a theme. They were all working so hard! They worked hard to cut out fat or carbs or sugar or calories and they were exercising more. Most were not losing weight or enough weight or they weren't coming back to see me.

I constantly heard: "Julie, you don't understand."

On the outside, I just nodded my head to show that I was emphatically listening. Inside, I thought, "What do you mean I don't understand? I have sat with literally hundreds of kids and families going through the same thing as you, and there are so many common themes, similar struggles, and experiences, feelings of shame, disappointment, fear, loneliness, sadness, and I've felt all those things. I totally understand. I totally get it."

A few times, I told people that I *did* understand, and it only took a few times for me to realize that was not the right way to go. They told me I didn't get it. I didn't.

I have always had a straight-sized body. I have never had to go to a special store to find clothes that fit me. If you lined up every one of my family, you would notice they all look like me.

Because I appreciate diet culture doesn't lift up only thin bodies, let me tell you about all of my identities. I am white, specifically European-American, cisgender, heterosexual, divorced, and raised as a Christian yet no longer practicing. I manage two chronic health conditions: migraine and insulin resistance.

While my life has ups and downs, I was born into a life of privilege. I've had lots of hard things happen in my life yet most have been easier for me because of my earth suit—the body you were born into.

I began connecting with my privileges as a pediatric dietitian. It was tough for me to make sense of them and continue to help people with different identities, so I pursued a master's degree in mental health counseling. I hoped this education would give me better tools to finally help people lose weight, get healthier, and feel better about themselves all along the way.

In my very first counseling class, I asked my professor, Dr. Spurgeon, "What do you say when a client says, 'You don't understand'?"

He instructed: "You tell them they are right. You don't. And ask them to help you understand."

Over the next few years, he also helped me understand my own life more. Understanding those privileges has helped me unpack my personal inherent and learned biases.

Since that master's degree, I've been doing a lot of listening and learning and unlearning. All the years earlier as a dietitian, when I was listening to my clients, I was listening through a different set of ears. Those ears had yet to begin to understand the privileges I was given.

After my graduate program, I was listening with different types of ears and yet I still was in this place where I wanted to be better prepared to help people to be healthier, *to fix them*. I wanted to help people lose weight and to feel better about themselves at the same time.

In my first job out of graduate school, I was able to do counseling and work as a dietitian. I first worked as an eating disorder dietitian and continued working with higher-weight kids and their families. It also included helping people prepare for gastric bypass surgery (also known as stomach amputation surgery—a term I learned from Marilyn Wann) and teaching classes that were provided by an unnamed medically supervised liquid diet company.

As I dove into this new work with eating disorders, it felt oddly familiar. This surprised me. I realized it was so normal to me because my clients with eating disorders—while counting calories, cutting fat or carbs or sugar, and/or exercising more—were feeling that same guilt, sadness, shame, fear, loneliness as the higher-weight kids.

Clients with eating disorders were experiencing the same negative emotions yet I was helping them prioritize healing. We strategized ways with clients with eating disorders to help them reconnect with and repair their relationship with food.

But folks in a higher-weight body, whether they were prepping for surgery or doing those medically supervised diets or were those dieting higher-weight kids, the shame was the same. Instead of helping them move away from the shame, I was the one pushing it. I wasn't prioritizing healing for *everyone*. I was distancing higher-weight people from their innate relationship with food and trying to teach them to distrust it.

Working with patients with eating disorders exposed me to countercultural philosophies that reject dieting, including intuitive eating, mindful eating, and Health at Every Size® approaches. I quickly devoured books on these non-diet topics. As I was learning, I would teach these healing practices to folks with eating disorders and then turn around and teach a weight-loss class.

I felt like such a fraud. My work suffered, and of course the boss noticed.

The moment everything changed

So this brings you and me to that Big Cry with my boss.

Before the cry, I recognized the world easily had sympathy for those with stereotypical lower-weight anorexia and bulimia and the torture they inflicted on their bodies. But my higher-weight clients, the children and their families, were being tortured by food, too. They ate the same restrictive food plans. They counted calories, cutting fat or carbs or sugar and exercising more. They categorized food as good or bad, they exercised a lot, or limited their intake to medically supervised diets.

Here's the kicker: I told the higher-weight people to try harder. I praised their commitment. I failed to recognize that, because of my privilege and fatphobia, my higher-weight clients were being tortured too.

I really, really cared for my higher-weight clients, and I realized shortly before the Big Cry that I was expecting my higher-weight clients to practice the very behaviors I called pathological and diseased in my lower-weight clients. I wasn't helping my clients. I was *harming* them.

I sat with people as they signed on the dotted line to amputate part of their stomach. I coached them how to say no to social invitations because of the food that was going to be served.

As I connected these dots, I couldn't sleep and I couldn't eat.

Alright, we finally get to the day of the Big Cry.

One of my first classes was a positive body image class for that unnamed diet company. And honestly, these classes were super easy to execute because there was an outline and script prepared for me. All I had to do was show up, push a mental play button, and go through the material. I didn't even have to think.

It was supposed to be a 30-minute class. Standing at the front of the classroom—in my thin, white body—my job was to guide higher-weight people on how to love their marginalized bodies but also on how to torture those same marginalized bodies because they were wrong.

The cognitive dissonance I experienced in that moment, standing in front of the class, was intolerable. I trembled, turning the script pages back and forth. Words literally wouldn't come out of my mouth. I was trying to hold together my values of helping without harming and helping people to lose weight. But they couldn't reside together in my brain any longer.

So I stopped.

The entire lesson lasted three minutes.

When my boss met with me (I have to say this woman was such a compassionate, kind person, and bore no blame for doing her job), she was disappointed and angry. She let me know that I had got a number of complaints—people had paid for a 30-minute class and I had shortchanged them by 27 minutes.

I proceeded to let her know about my ethical dilemma. Through my sobs, I said I could no longer contribute to this harm and place people on diets because it felt immoral.

I wanted to help people repair their relationship with food yet I was only giving that option to a select few.

I wanted to promote health but could no longer contribute to the *harm*. I told her weight loss is not a behavior and expecting it was proof of my fatphobia. I wasn't able to help put people on diets anymore.

Very kindly and firmly, she let me know I needed to do all of the different parts of my job as I was hired to do.

So I quit.

Before you give me any high fives, remember the privileges I experienced are not accessible to all. I had just gotten married and had this opportunity to join my husband's healthcare plan. We had the financial stability and flexibility to give me time to open a private practice.

Many healthcare providers right now are working a job with the same ethical dilemmas. They are still in the position, not because they don't want to quit, but because it's the only way to make ends meet or it's the only job in the area, or they need to keep their health insurance. I'm sending compassion to anyone in that place.

Finding my way using intuitive eating

I started my private practice in January 2005, just days after quitting my job. I specialized in eating disorders as well as helping people recover from chronic dieting using an intuitive eating framework.

Evelyn Tribole and Elyse Resch wrote the revolutionary book *Intuitive Eating* in 1995.[1] As the book evolved through several editions, it provided me with a framework to help clients quit dieting and make peace with food.

As the months turned to years, I was one of few dietitians in my small town offering non-diet nutrition. While I quickly felt competent in helping people recover from eating disorders, I felt less prepared to help people with chronic conditions move toward these non-diet approaches.

In particular, many clients with polycystic ovary syndrome (PCOS) contacted me at rock bottom. They described decades' worth of diet attempts that brought only chaos, bingeing, and self-loathing. They were exhausted. They exercised more than anyone believed. They were gaining weight but eating such minuscule amounts that doctors thought they were lying.

Clients desperately wanted to heal their relationship with food, yet it felt out of reach because of their medical diagnosis. Healthcare providers led each person to believe they had to eat less (especially carbs and sugar) and move more because of these chronic conditions.

Have you felt that desperation, too? Have you heard of intuitive eating and thought, "It won't work for me because I have to diet for my health"?

In these early stages of my private practice, I knew diets didn't work for most people, so why would they work for most people with PCOS or another diagnosis?

Do you *have* to diet?

I still remember my first client with PCOS after the Big Cry. Sitting on my green couch, Matilda told me through tears about all the diets she had done only to feel like a failure. She did everything doctors told her to do to bring back regular menstrual cycles and lessen the classic PCOS intense carbohydrate cravings.

I jotted down all the diets she tried—low or no carb, WW, keto, paleo, low calorie—that overpromised on results yet underdelivered on outcomes.

Instead of feeling more energetic, she was painfully tired and constantly thinking about food. She brought old food records in case I didn't believe how little she had eaten while on each diet.

Flipping through countless smudged and grease-stained pages, I saw how "compliant" Matilda was with each diet. Looking at each dated entry, I could feel the hope coming from the page as she began each diet. She meticulously recorded eating times, amounts, feelings, and events. I saw the math work as she calculated macros, eating times, or calories— whatever variable was in vogue when it came to a particular diet.

Looking closer, I could see the tear stains, too.

How heartbreaking to seek guidance on a medical condition only to be prescribed something that was just about guaranteed not to work?

I sat, holding all of Matilda's journals, speechless. In the easy chair, I tried to take it all in. She had tried to manage her PCOS symptoms and lose weight for most of her life. What could I recommend that would be different?

Lost in my thoughts, Matilda squeaked out a barely audible question: "Do you believe me? I have tried all the diets and none has worked. I promise I was not doing anything wrong."

It was easy for me to believe Matilda. She wasn't the first person in a higher-weight body diet their life away with no outcomes to speak of except a complicated relationship with food and body shame. I paused before answering. Instead of enthusiastically yelling *yes!* I wanted to know more.

"What makes you ask, Matilda?"

What Matilda said next has been repeated now at least a thousand times on that same green couch. Healthcare providers told her there was no way she was actually eating that little or exercising that much— if she were doing all those things, she would've lost weight by now and her cycles would've normalized. Sometimes they didn't even ask Matilda what diet she had been following and merely recommended higher calorie amounts or carb restrictions significantly looser than those Matilda was already torturing herself with.

Healthcare providers always assumed she was eating too much or spending her time too sedentarily. I have a feeling the word "noncompliance" was written in her chart notes because her weight loss wasn't going as the provider planned.

I told Matilda what I want to tell you: *I believe you and I am sorry others haven't.*

You have tried hard enough, even if you have dieted only once or are lucky enough never to have dieted before.

No matter what you weigh or what you have been diagnosed with—including but not limited to diabetes, PCOS, fatty liver disease, high cholesterol or any other chronic condition added to the Diet Cures It bucket—you are enough as you are.

When I met with Matilda, I was a new non-diet dietitian. I knew in every cell of my body that diets didn't work, but my instinct was to prescribe a diet to someone with something like PCOS.

What about their high insulin levels? Their risk for diabetes? Heart disease?

Could I trust intuitive eating even then?

I walked over to my bookshelf stuffed with all my college texts and more recent self-help books. I pulled out what we dietitians often refer to as "The Krause Book," the 6.5-pound tome that integrates human physiology, biochemistry, and dietetics.[2] As a young professional, I often grabbed it to look up information that was not yet readily available. I hoped it would give me something to hang my new non-diet dietitian hat on.

Unfortunately, one little measly paragraph described nutrition interventions for people with PCOS. It was at the same time absolute and ambiguous. It read: "Treat [people] with PCOS like you would with diabetes. Teach carbohydrate counting and how to manage weight."

I closed it with disgust and turned back to Matilda.

In that moment, I knew I was on my own. Before, I had relied on evidence-based practice written by my senior colleagues to direct my clinical practice. But this was when I realized that they had failed me. Instead of relying on *just* scholarly journal articles, I needed to also rely on Matilda.

I told her I had come to appreciate how diets harm most people and that her experiences were more the norm than the exception. Sadly, eating less and focusing on weight loss were the only nutrition interventions studied. We literally had nothing else to go on.

But we could still try something different.

I was frank about my novice non-diet skills and interest in finding another way with her to live with her chronic condition. Did Matilda want to try intuitive eating instead?

I am grateful she said yes.

Because of Matilda and thousands of others, I have witnessed people moving away from diets and towards improving their physical and emotional health. Gathering their outcomes and tools that helped, I can firmly say you too do not have to diet.

If you have tried to quit dieting, it may have felt impossible, especially if you live with diabetes or another chronic condition. We are brought up to believe that each bite can either kill us or cure us.[3] What an impossible wedge for you! To have all that power and yet feel powerless when each diet ends in failure—you must be exhausted.

Most non-diet tools are misunderstood. All-or-nothing cultural food beliefs block access to your healing, to finding your Food Voice.

Your Food Voice is an internal system you were born with to communicate when to eat, how much, and what choices to consume based on what is available. This communication may be through body awareness like hunger, fullness, fatigue, mood, or satisfaction. This communication may also be through thoughts and feelings or guided by structured self-care techniques. Your Food Voice will be unique to the individual yet always flexible, kind, and nurturing. Its primary function is to help the person prioritize eating enough. It is a *knowing* with an unconditional permission for food yet compassionate when outside circumstances block access.

Finding *your* Food Voice will help you bring all of your food and body wishes together. Dump them on a table and lovingly sift through them all. As you read this book, I hope you give yourself the space to examine each and every one. There may be some that you decide you no longer want to keep, some you want to put on a figurative shelf as a maybe, and others you want to pull even closer.

This work will bring intense emotions including:

- joy
- happiness
- peace
- sadness
- grief
- anger
- comfort.

Some will feel expected yet others will surprise you. Many conflicting emotions will happen at the same time. None of them is wrong.

Reconnecting with your Food Voice is hard work and it is good work. It is messy and beautiful. It is concrete and a cluster. I cannot spell out exactly what your Food Voice is, and while that may be disappointing, it is on purpose.

I promise I will share with you why you haven't been doing it wrong all along with food but have been given many distracting, harmful, and unnecessary eating instructions. Finding your Food Voice will help you identify what's disconnecting you from knowing how to eat and will repair your dusty internal compass so you can stop dieting forever.

Here's our plan

Our food culture has conflated health and worth with weight. What if you wrote a letter to Food? Put pen to paper and hash or thrash out your love/hate relationship and Food's undeserving power. The details may go back years, to your first childhood diet as you tried to fit in. In this letter, examine your dusty Food beliefs and wonder which should go in the trash, which are for others, and which remain in your heart. What if you wrote this all down and Food wrote back to you?

I invite you to write as many letters to Food as you need. Each chapter in this book begins with a letter to Food and ends with a letter Food writes back. While recovering from dieting is messy and nonlinear, I hope each letter back from Food helps you decide your next steps.

Here is Food's letter back to me:

Dear Concerned Dietitian,

Your letter is right on time. All of us—vegetables, fruits, proteins, carbs, sugars, fats, desserts, candy, and everyone else—we got together recently and talked about the smoother days ... the days when we were all a normal part of a person's life all together. We have a tough time keeping up with who's in the "good" category and who is in the "bad." Sometimes, one of us is both! Concerned Dietitian, we would love to give input and insight into this important topic of food for healing, health, and wellbeing. We are *tired* of the dieting industry confusing *all* of us, and keeping people from enjoying us. We will treat each Dear Food letter with kindness and respect. This will be tough work and important work for everyone. We look forward to these next steps.

Love,
Food

References

1 Tribole, E., & Resch, E. (2020). *Intuitive Eating: A Revolutionary Anti-diet Approach*. St. Martin's Essentials.
2 Mahan, L. K., and Raymond, J. L. (2016). *Krause's Food & the Nutrition Care Process*, 14th edn. Saunders.
3 Tribole and Resch, *Intuitive Eating*.

2

Seduction

Dear Food,

It's never been easy for you and me. I watched as my younger sisters growing up never thought twice about you, happily eating what they wanted, as much as they wanted, whenever they wanted. They grew into normal bodies, well fueled for taking on academic and athletic endeavors. Food was food.

You and I, though? Not so much. In third grade, when in an attempt to "help me," my mom encouraged me to eat a plain baked potato with salsa. But, just me. Not my sisters, not the rest of the family. It was the first lesson that you and I couldn't be friends, that our relationship was different—strained, fraught, always at odds.

One of the biggest problems is I was a "good girl." I still am. I did what I was told to do—what my mom told me to eat or not eat, what was "appropriate" based on the food pyramid in school, or what the latest diet craze was.

After three decades of this battle, I'm covered in scars of damage seen and unseen. Stretch marks and depression, fat rolls and anxiety. Each time, I tried harder and harder, but it never worked. It wasn't just my own disappointment that I was contending with—I saw it on my mom's face, on my grandma's face. Their own struggles with body size, now showing up in their tears and frustration and sadness for me, because I was not able to "achieve my goal." But was it ever really my goal to begin with? Food, I didn't start this mess. But I believed in it. And now, try as hard as I might, I can't seem to shake that feeling.

Possibly the saddest thing? I look back at photos of that young girl, and I see how wrong they all were. Oh, but to have a time machine so I could go back and tell my younger self that she is beautiful and perfect and worthy of you, Food. To protect her from all that was stolen and end the war before it even started.

Alas, here we are, Food. I'm short a time travel machine and fucking tired of the constant battles, so I'm left to reconcile and grieve for what we've lost or what I wish could have been. Now, though, I see you were never the enemy. The battle is not with you—it never was. I could place the blame and anger on my mom, and her mom, and so on and so forth. But that still doesn't seem fair—they didn't choose this hurt either. Instead, I take on the arduous work to heal, to break the cycle, to choose peace. It may not come easy, but now I see our relationship is worth it. More importantly, I'm worth it.

Wishing you love and peace,
Your friend, Kim

How long have you been stuck trying different diets? How many have you been on? When was the first one?

Do you ever think back to the very first time the diet idea popped into your head? How did it get there?

I remember speaking with Rae (they/them) about their first diet that started in kindergarten. The pediatrician noted how their weight had jumped up from the year before and scolded Rae's mom for not teaching mealtime discipline. She instructed Mom to stop giving Rae seconds. The pediatrician jokingly mentioned eating differently would make everyone jealous of Rae and want to be their friend.

Five-year-old Rae knew eating less would be hard, but the payoff was high. The doctor promised popularity in exchange for dieting. Dieting would even make Rae's mom a better parent.

Forty years later, the seed planted in Rae's mind became an orchard of shame, chaos, disconnection, desperation, and self-loathing. We charted Rae's roller-coaster diet history spanning four decades; each life milestone Rae remembered their weight and the diet getting them there. There were common themes each time Rae started a diet: a renewed hopefulness that this was the one.

Rae told me in our first session they felt trapped in a diet trap and wanted to get out. But just like many people, dieting was the only way Rae knew how to take care of their eating decisions.

If you have been dieting a long time, too, not dieting may feel impossible or even immoral. How did dieting get to be ingrained as the only way to eat? After a long history of dieting, why is it hard to stop?

Consider this metaphor. If you have ever returned a rental car, you may recall the pointed spikes that allow you to move forward yet not back. Once you get to a certain point, there is a moment when you can no longer reverse out again. You are trapped moving in one direction. Diets have the same moving forward requirement.

If you are like Rae and can't imagine a life without a set of food rules, you are in the Diet Trap. Your brain is stuck in the rental car garage and hit that place of no going back. The Diet Trap lays hold of people within just a few diets, and many stay stuck in this cycle for decades. Some never get out again and will always be ruled by what to eat and what not to eat. Food will always take up too much mental energy and they will be guilt-ridden. But it doesn't have to be that way, and I will show you a way out.

Your Diet Trap resembles a never-ending roundabout that goes like this:

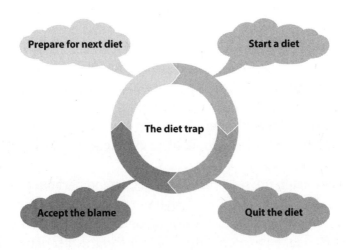

There are systems at play that push you into your first Diet Trap cycle, and even more systems that keep you stuck. My promise to you:

understanding which systems keep you in the cycle will help you break away from your own personal Diet Trap.

Life in the Diet Trap can feel like a big failure. One woman once told me that, with each diet ending, she failed three times: she was a quitter, she didn't lose weight, and she was still fat. The Diet Trap convinced her that losing weight and controlling food was the only way to live. The reality, though, is that, for many years now, you have been a successful human. You have managed all the eating decisions that have helped you stay alive since your very first breath. Even with all this practice, why do so many of us have doubts we can handle food decisions? Why does *not* dieting feel like breaking a commandment?

We live in a culture that trains us to distrust our bodies and leads us to believe we need to follow outside orders to decide every bite we put in our mouth. It doesn't matter how long the weight loss takes, how ineffective the diet is, or how much pain it creates. Diets have been downloaded into our brains and bodies without our consent as the default eating setting. Which systems contribute to this cryptic computer virus download? This chapter will help you gain clarity on the specific systems impacting your food history. First of all, though, let's learn a little more about Rae.

Like other chronic dieters before them, Rae explained to me the laundry list of what they could and could not eat. They said: "I should be eating more vegetables. I should not be eating as many processed foods. I must not eat after 7, or wait at least 12 hours between dinner and breakfast, or else... or else what I don't know."

All of Rae's *shoulds* led them toward a learned shame, guilt, and distrust of their own ability to make food decisions. Rae was born knowing how and how much to eat through a system that was their own. Rae didn't need these *shoulds*.

You don't need the *shoulds* either. They've disconnected you, too, from that *knowing*.

Rae kept dieting for years and felt pinned down by the Diet Trap. When I asked what kept them starting each new diet—even after decades of proof that diets weren't working for them—Rae responded, "I feel so good when I am dieting, at least in the beginning."

Do you relate?

The Diet Trap eventually becomes a perpetual seduction. It tricks us into believing a fantasy that in reality does not exist. Besides keeping us tortured with food, this seduction distracts us from the systems behind it all. I refer to this seduction as the *I-Should-Eat* script. It overpromises the simplicity of weight loss and under-delivers on its guarantee for lasting thinness and all that comes from it.

Everyone gets seduced by the *I-Should-Eat* script in their lifetime. When you get introduced to it depends on factors including how close you are to being thin, white, and cisgender, how much power you have in the world, and whether you are susceptible to an eating disorder. But who is doing the seducing? The diet industry.

In 2023, the U.S. weight loss market made $75 billion.[1] The market includes meal replacements, health clubs, weight loss medications, supplements, diet drinks, technology companies, and anything related to making you look and eat a particular way. Sylvester Graham, of Graham Crackers fame, started the U.S. dieting trend in the 1830s.[2] He was a Presbyterian minister who thought eating certain flours would morally corrupt us. His solution? A new flour he sold. Over the next almost 200 years, diet recommendations infiltrated popular magazines, healthcare recommendations, and public policy. They are now everywhere from what makes up a complete breakfast, to what solids to start feeding your baby, to what is acceptable to give your dog. All the recommendations focus on making sure we (or our pets) are not eating too much.

At least 45 million Americans diet every year. Don't be fooled into thinking that diet companies care about our health. The diet industry is a money-making machine that only suggests food, exercise, and weight decisions in order to keep their pockets lined.

The diet industry and escalating eating disorders

Before you skip this section: eating disorders have a role in your complicated food history even if you have never been diagnosed with one. Appreciating the *I-Should-Eat* script connection to eating disorders will help you find your way out of the Diet Trap.

I remember getting an email from Keisha looking for a way to schedule an appointment for her daughter without a doctor's referral.

She explained in the email that she was concerned about her daughter's eating habits even though the pediatrician wasn't because her weight had been stable. When we met, Keisha cried while describing how little her teen daughter Traci ate and how depressed Traci's mood became with less food. Keisha, who described her own body as fat, said her daughter's health class focused on healthy eating and got Traci invested in not gaining too much weight. Even though her eating habits drastically changed, Traci's weight did not. This appeared to only fuel Traci's food restrictions. On paper, it was easy to see that Traci was suffering from anorexia nervosa and needed medical attention urgently. Keisha and I knew her pediatrician was not concerned because Traci was Black and higher weight.

Do you picture a certain person when you imagine someone diagnosed with an eating disorder? I did for a long time and that person was usually a white, very thin, affluent teenager. Know that the majority of people with eating disorders go undiagnosed. They are also higher weight and not white. Income level has no impact on whether someone experiences an eating disorder, just on whether they get treatment or not. If you do not fit the eating disorder stereotype, and feel stuck in a Diet Trap, there's a high likelihood you have experienced an eating disorder. You could still be right now.

Even if you don't meet the criteria now or ever for an eating disorder, know dieting is not normal eating. Dieting is disordered eating, and it changes how your brain thinks about food. Warning: if you want to argue with me on this one, I will die on this hill. Even without an eating disorder diagnosis, life within the Diet Trap causes suffering and negatively impacts your life.

The diet industry's canary

Before savvy gas detection equipment existed, miners took canaries and other birds down into the mine with them. A singing bird signaled safe air. Silent birds meant the air was dangerous. This system helped keep miners safe because birds would become unconscious and die from toxic fumes before humans. The coal miners knew as long as the birds were singing, they were safe, too.

Folks with eating disorders are our metaphorical canary in our toxic diet industry culture cave. If you have an eating disorder, we have ignored your struggle for too long. We have allowed diets to fester and permeate our thoughts and behaviors, and that has devastated you first. We have minimized diet recommendations as harmless so they are flippantly given out at doctor appointments and at the dinner table.

Diet culture is at toxic levels. Only now we are all at risk.

Back when I first started working with folks with eating disorders, I noticed each client maintained a mental list dictating what they could and could not eat. It was rigid and delivered like a stern order. Often, the list changed with the nutrition headlines of the moment, but the orders were always delivered like a sweaty, angry coach with a loud whistle. One strategy I used to help people decipher their eating disorder thoughts and behaviors was to name their eating disorder demands as if coming from an outside entity. Many chose "Ed" for this angry coach. Naming Ed helped to discern between harmful thoughts versus ones they wanted to focus on for recovery. Separating out these rigid rules helped my clients and me distinguish between directions that were helping with healing and those that were not. It felt like removing big heavy rocks off their innate Food Voice.

Whenever clients with eating disorders did not follow Ed's mandates, clients would describe feeling bad. Bad ended up being coded language for buckets of shame and layers of unworthiness.

Even when I worked with clients without diagnosed eating disorders, I found they had a similar whistleblowing coach spewing hatred and shame to try to motivate behavior change. Even without a diagnosed condition, folks coming to see me so they could eat more healthily or manage a chronic condition had that same rigid list barking in their head.

Many of us feel bad about our eating, and unworthy, too. Big heavy rocks start to pile up blocking us from that *knowing* how to instinctively manage our eating decisions. Looking into your own post-diet buckets of shame, what do you see? When a diet ends, do you feel like a failure because you are not an after picture?

One thing that appears to temporarily yet significantly lessen those bad feelings is yet another new diet.

When you start a food plan, do you feel a spark of hopefulness? Do you start to picture life after the diet has delivered on its promises?

Don't be fooled: even if it is not called a diet, it has the same power. You could call this new hopeful plan a lifestyle change or just eating healthily. The words may be different yet the seduction is the same.

We can learn from folks with eating disorders. They experienced the toxic levels from the diet industry before everyone else. They experienced the first seductive yet toxic fumes from the *I-Should-Eat* script. Now we are still breathing in the same noxious air yet can't find the exits. The way out? Let's shine a light on your version of the *I-Should-Eat* script.

Your *I-Should-Eat* script

Wrapped up into a pretty package with a big, blousy bow, the diet industry delivers a predictable sequence of emotions to lead you into the Diet Trap. While stuck on that roundabout, the script outlines a simple to-do list promising to meet your needs. So subtle in the beginning, the *I-Should-Eat* script quickly evolves into mind control while cleverly avoiding incriminating itself, and distracting you from the real villain.

You got seduced not because you are broken or have been doing it wrong. Rather, you have been lied to by the real villain within the diet industry: oppressive systems. They include racism, homophobia, ableism, xenophobia, misogyny, classism, transphobia, healthism, weight-based stigma, and other systems that keep white supremacy as the majority power. We know white supremacy, as defined by the *Merriam-Webster's Collegiate Dictionary*, as the "belief that the white race is inherently superior to other races and that white people should have control over people of other races." It also states that white supremacy is "the social, economic, and political systems that collectively enable white people to maintain power over people of other races."[3] White supremacy upholds that the perfect body is:

- white
- cisgender
- able-bodied
- heterosexual
- thin.

These systems direct you to follow specific orders through laws, customs, and practices that have evolved over centuries. These orders appear to have the good intention of keeping you relevant and compliant. The further you are from a white cisgender thin body, the more the script seems to be keeping you physically safe.

Before you go any further, a gentle heads-up. This next bit of this chapter will help you notice the sly workings of the *I-Should-Eat* script. Know that once you see it, you can't unsee it. Like my Big Cry, you too will have a before and after that's altogether unlike those side-by-side Instagram posts. You won't appear different yet *everything* will change. I appreciate this will be hard work but I promise the outcome will be powerful. You will begin to connect the dots that you aren't doing it wrong but have been given the wrong tools. Tools that hurt you and keep you in the Diet Trap.

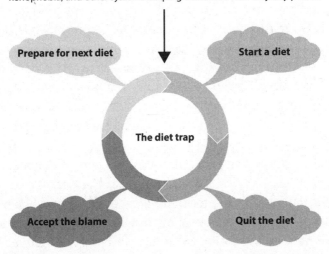

Oppressive systems
Racism, weight bias, sexism, transphobia, ableism, homophobia, xenophobia, and other systems keeping whiteness with majority power.

The *I-Should-Eat* scripts give you hope

Diets and preparing for them give the notion things will be all right *soon*. Rae told me about the times they tried to not diet using the non-diet concept of intuitive eating but that eating then felt overwhelming and chaotic. Not dieting exhausted their brain because of all the food decisions constantly tapping them on the shoulder. The brain needed to know:

- When to eat?
- What to prepare?
- How to prepare it?
- How much to eat?
- How fast to eat it?
- Who to eat it with?
- Should there be leftovers?
- How hungry do I need to be?
- How full do I need to be when finished?
- What if I am not hungry?
- What if I am hungry for more than I made?
- What do I even want to eat?

Not only are these questions begging for answers every day, but hundreds of times throughout the day.

No wonder just the act of deciding to embark on a new diet relaxed and calmed Rae. Instead of being exhausted and doubtful, a fresh diet decision feels powerful because you don't have to make as many decisions. It feels easier. Your head feels clear for the first time in a long time. Diet relief is dose dependent on how much chaos you have with food—the more you can gain in life from a diet success, the more the adrenaline rush.

A new diet plan feels like a reassuring hug from a trusted kind mentor who promises to scoop you up and put you on the next right path. "Put your worries away," your script says. "You can relax now because I have a plan. Just follow these simple eating directions."

The first few days or weeks after you embark on a diet can give off electric sparks of excitement. Rae told me they felt this because they always got encouragement from well-meaning friends and family. Folks would notice different foods in Rae's lunches or ordering something different when out to eat. The amount of people compelled to comment on a person's new diet blows me away. Even more, people in power seem especially compelled to give new diet high fives. When else do bosses, mothers, pastors, and doctors all notice a behavior change?

No wonder a new diet is so exciting.

Have you felt this before? Can you feel it now?

That is a diet's first seduction every time you start one—keeping you in the Diet Trap.

How *I-Should-Eat* scripts fuel the fantasy

Diets promise more than weight loss. Check out the history of every diet industry product and you will see this, too. Diet company advertisements promise you:

- health
- long life
- acceptance
- confidence
- peace
- relevance
- you will be the source of envy
- you will be seen
- belonging
- a romantic partner
- you will love yourself
- permanent solutions.

Rae was told that dieting and the associated weight loss would make them more popular! As a young child that was all the bait needed to get them started obeying a list of allowed foods and swearing off those that were not.

Even if you were older than Rae when you started dieting, diets promised you outcomes. What have diets promised you?

While the promises listed above have a hold, there are others often overlooked but which are important. If you hold identities that have been historically marginalized, diets also promise:

- safety (from microaggressions or violence)
- access (to comfortable seating, healthcare, surgical options, reproductive medicine, gender-affirming care, etc.)
- dignity (to get pictures taken only with consent, eat a meal without ridicule, permission for pleasure, etc.)
- respect (taken seriously for job promotions, academic options, etc.).

I appreciate this is not an exhaustive list. What have I missed? What are some of the foundational human needs that diets (and their weight-loss outcomes) promise you?

How *I-Should-Eat* scripts promise outcomes

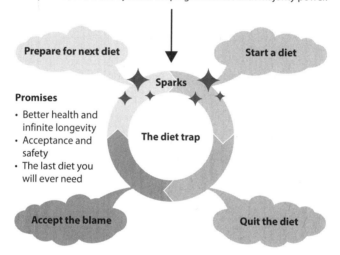

Oppressive systems

Racism, weight bias, sexism, transphobia, ableism, homophobia, xenophobia, and other systems keeping whiteness with majority power.

Prepare for next diet

Start a diet

Sparks

Promises
- Better health and infinite longevity
- Acceptance and safety
- The last diet you will ever need

The diet trap

Accept the blame

Quit the diet

Diets promise better health

My first dietitian job (years before the Big Cry) was on a cardiac step-down unit at a big teaching hospital. My patients had just experienced some kind of scary life-altering event like a heart attack and had recently stepped down from intensive care. Those transferred to my floor were lucky since many people never lived to see life outside of the ICU. By the time I met with them, they were breathing huge sighs of relief and ready to go home.

I stood in the way between the scary hospital and the comforts of home. Discharge papers would not be signed until each patient attended my Heart Healthy Discharge Class. I taught them how to increase fruit and vegetable intake and which foods to avoid to promote cardiovascular health. I remember some patients furiously writing notes whereas others snoozed with loud snores.

Those awake in class probably took home a message like "If you eat right, you can avoid coming back to this hellscape. You and you alone have the power to prevent another heart attack."

At this stage of my career, even though I had not yet met a non-diet dietitian, I doubted the power of my diet instruction at these classes. Even then I connected with the idea that the diet promise sounded a bit too slick.

Diet messages cradle us most when we fear death or disability. Diets like the heart-healthy ones I taught in those discharge classes promise better health, prolonged ability, and longer lifespan. Of course, you don't have to experience a heart attack to fear one. I remember seeing this close to home when my kids were taught at school how to fear foods because of their connotation with diabetes and heart disease. We are taught early on how every bite contributes to our health *or* demise. Evelyn Tribole, coauthor of *Intuitive Eating*, says, "We are taught that every bite of food will either kill us or cure us." Diets promise to take care of us just as long as we follow their list of stipulations. With that spark of hopefulness we get when starting a new diet plan, the health promise acts like the oxygen feeding the flames of your diet mojo. Those patients furiously scribbling notes in my Heart Healthy Discharge Class believed my words were the Gospel according to Those-Who-Know-Better. Following the preacher (me) would keep them out of the ICU and maybe just maybe keep them alive forever. Diets promise eternal life, even though none of us is getting out of here alive.

Diets promise this is the last diet you will need

With every new diet, Rae thought it would be the last one they would need to start. Those patients just minutes from discharge writing verbatim notes in my Heart Healthy Discharge Class thought my food lists were the last they would need to take. Part of each diet promise includes a guarantee it will be The One.

I speak with very few people who are just starting their very first diet because most have been dieting for years already. If diets don't end up working, why do folks keep starting them?

That hopeful spark keeps luring us back to dieting and somehow the diet industry has convinced us their diet will finally be the one to work.

Whether it is WW (previously known as Weight Watchers), Optavia (formerly Medifast), a medical weight-loss clinic, GLP-1 agonists, or a dietitian selling a program—they all promise they have the secret to lasting weight loss.

Rae told me how, with each heartbreaking end to a diet, part of them felt okay because another diet was an option. Each time, Rae convinced themselves that it was user error that had brought about failure and that another new diet would finally set them free. So while they felt hopeless about that diet, the promise of a new one strung Rae along, convincing them to keep on trying.

When WW didn't work, Rae knew they could try switching up macros. When counting macros didn't end well, they read about intermittent fasting. After intermittent fasting led to binge eating, Rae thought keto would be the diet to work. When keto fell flat, their doctor recommended GLP-1s. Can you relate? With each weight-loss promise broken, another guaranteed silver bullet awaits, microdosing the hope that keeps us from seeing the Diet Trap's exit.

The rotating diet options strengthen the diet industry. Switching around what is on your *I-Should-Eat* script provides enough variability to keep you hopeful that the changes will provide the lasting benefit. Changing around what to calculate or focus on shifts the focus away from the diet's failings and instead keeps you the dieter looking forward, not back (remember those rental car return spikes!), convinced you are almost there and the next diet will work.

Your *I-Should-Eat* scripts distract you from key facts

Distraction #1: Diets do not work

The diet industry waves its metaphorical hands, distracting us from weight science research. Confirmed many times over, we have yet to discover a way for someone to lose weight that is sustainable and health promoting for most people in the long term. In a nutshell: zero diets have been found to work long-term. I want to reassure you: you and your body on diets have always been part of the norm rather than the anomaly.

I hear you all the way from here saying diets *did work* for you until you stopped dieting. If diets worked, why do you need to keep going on them?

Something we need to clarify is what I mean by the word *work*. I define working diets to have these mandatory ingredients:

- They are doable for the majority of the people who go on the diet.
- They promote physical health in the short and long term.
- They promote positive mental health in the short and long term.
- Weight loss must be maintained for the majority of participants at least five years later.

Using these ingredients, no diet studies have generated long-term weight loss results for the majority of participants. According to review studies, long-term follow-up studies say most people will regain their weight loss regardless of whether they continue with the program or not.[4] A National Institute of Health Panel of experts determined one-third to two-thirds of weight lost from dieting is regained within one year and almost all within five years.[5]

Long-term review of weight science research also finds one-third to two-thirds of dieters regain more weight than they lost on their diets. The researchers summarize: there is little support for the idea that diets lead to lasting weight loss or health benefits.

Distraction #2: The pursuit of weight loss worsens health

Part of diet's seductive fantasy minimizes the risk of pursuing weight loss. What's the big deal if someone wants to lose five or ten pounds just to fit into a different size and feel more confident? Or even more, what if someone is in a very large body? Isn't it harmful for you to not help people lose weight? Isn't that promoting harm in doing that?

There is a real risk of dieting that I want you to know about that comes from weight changes. Stuck in the Diet Trap, most people lose weight only to gain it back. Research has already established this as the predictable norm, and every dieter should expect weight regain back to their starting weight. Some people will regain more than they lost in the first place. This up-and-down weight change is called weight cycling. Weight cycling causes a number of health conditions as well as reduces how many calories we need to eat to maintain weight.

A large body of literature has connected weight cycling directly with poor health including:

higher mortality	higher blood sugar
higher risk of osteoporotic fractures	higher insulin levels
	high blood pressure
gallstone attacks	chronic inflammation
loss of muscle tissue	some forms of cancer.

Framingham Heart Study examined mortality and morbidity in more than 5,000 individuals over a 32-year period. The researchers found weight cycling was strongly linked to overall mortality as well as mortality and morbidity related to coronary heart disease for both men and women.[6]

In the ERFORT Study conducted in Germany, 505 middle-aged men were grouped into weight categories of stable obese, stable nonobese, weight loss, weight gain, and weight fluctuations. Among these groupings only the weight fluctuation category was associated with mortality over the 15-year follow-up period. And even more, the stable obese category was not linked to higher risk of early death compared to the stable nonobese category.[7] Research using data from the NHANES study found that women with a weight cycling history (39% of the sample) gained more weight over time and engaged in less physical activity but more binge eating than their non-cycling peers.[8]

Weight science research also tells us the act of dieting leads to decreased energy needs. The Biggest Loser study illuminated this dieting risk. From this study we are able to gather that a person at a higher weight who has gone on and off diets will need a lower calorie amount to maintain their weight than someone at the same exact weight who has never dieted.[9]

I appreciate taking this all in makes things messier. The weight science research doesn't show evidence of a way to sustainably lose weight, yet a smaller body could improve access to travel, jobs, education, and health care options. It may even keep you safer from violence. What you do with your body is your choice, and that choice may include still wanting to pursue weight loss.

If that is your next step, please consider gaining full informed consent. Keep in mind these key points if you choose to continue to focus on weight loss:

- It probably won't lead to long-term weight loss.
- It probably will lower your calories needed to maintain your weight.
- It puts you at higher risk for mortality.
- It raises your risk for hypertension, higher blood sugar, inflammation, binge eating, and low self-concept.

Diets don't work for most people long-term so they probably won't for you either. Instead, dieting will probably lead to weight cycling, and this yo-yo effect is known to be a risk factor for health problems.

Instead of the diet decreasing a risk factor as promised by the diet industry, it is just adding another.

Living in a world prioritizing thin, white, able bodies makes the move away from diets more complicated than just not dieting. As you move through this book, please be compassionate with your choices when it comes to deciding what to eat and how to move your body. Be curious about what makes you decide to pursue weight loss. Keep the research in mind in case you weight cycle or experience anything negative after dieting. The shame or blame you feel doesn't belong to you: it belongs to the diet industry and oppressive systems.

Distraction #3: Weight loss is not a behavior

What about people who *do* maintain weight loss? What are they doing?

While I was working with clients with eating disorders, I noticed a small percentage kept their weight lower using extreme behaviors. While their weight was lower, physical and emotional health suffered. Relationships were strained from the rigid food rules. My clients' partners started to be able to predict irritable moods caused by the restrictive intake. Over time, physical health problems emerged, too, including missed periods, brittle bones, weakened heart muscles, hair loss, and lower libido.

My higher-weight clients (those with and without eating disorders) used identical behaviors yet just didn't get the same weight-loss results. Seeing this over and over again helped me to appreciate weight loss is not a behavior. No one can predict whether a diet will lead to weight loss, but we can predict it will eventually lead to worsened emotional and physical health.

Distraction #4: Diets pathologize normal food preoccupation

Paul (he/him) emailed me after listening to a *Find Your Food* podcast episode on food addiction. In this episode I bluntly state I don't believe food can be addicting. While I won't argue with someone referring to themselves as a food addict, I have yet to work with someone who continues to call themselves one after they stop dieting.

Paul wrote in his email that he would be the first to convince me he is a food addict. With the way food companies add sugar and salt and his weakness for potato chips after a stressful work day, he knew he would prove to me I was wrong. Whenever he had cookies and chips in his house, the food noise in his head was so loud he HAD to eat them. He could never keep them in the house ever again.

During Paul's first meetings we reviewed his extensive relationship with food. I discovered that his father was diagnosed with type 2 diabetes when Paul was in seventh grade and his mother painstakingly tried to create a home mirroring current diabetes guidelines. Before the diabetes diagnosis, his family had a variety of foods available including cookies for afterschool snacks and a candy drawer. Potato chips were a mainstay in the pantry which he was allowed to get food from whenever hungry. Once his dad was diagnosed with diabetes, fun foods like cookies, chips, and candies were not allowed to be in the home. Paul was told this was now a matter of life or death. Everyone had to ask before eating something, and he recalled getting yelled at whenever his mom would hear him try to sneak the pantry door open.

Weight loss started to be a central part of the family conversations. His mom didn't want his dad to be the only one dieting so she included the whole family. Paul's mom decided eating healthily and trying to lose a little weight was good for everyone.

Years later, Paul recalled getting through law-school all-night study sessions with coffee and a particular salty potato chip brand. He told me the crunching helped him stay awake and deal with the stress. It also helped him stay focused, which he said was important since he had been diagnosed with attention deficit hyperactivity disorder while in college. He nostalgically described the giant chocolate chip cookies he ate while relaxing after staying up all night; he would buy them after studying from the coffee shop near the library.

Paul told me in great detail the reason why he picked this particular chocolate chip cookie. The sweet-to-salt ratio, the crunchy outside and the soft middle, and the bonus of when it was still warm from the oven.

During the day, Paul carried on his mother's eating recommendations—he told me he was "good" at eating healthy during the day, so much so that he rewarded himself with potato chips and chocolate chip cookies at the end of it. He learned that if he kept these fun foods at home he would devour them in one sitting. Instead, he developed a ritual of eating these foods only while studying and never bringing them home. He did this so much that, whenever he opened a bag of potato chips, his mind knew it was time to get to work.

He carried these study rituals throughout law school yet stopped abruptly once working at a law firm. He was known as the health nut in the office, bringing salads to eat at his desk while everyone else ordered takeout. Paul loved being known as the only lawyer in the firm who was a healthy eater. I could see him beaming with pride.

Things started to unravel when he could no longer keep certain foods around him. He started dating his now spouse, Gene (she/they), a few years after law school. When they started living together, his partner would include potato chips during a grocery run. When the chips were in the house, Paul could not stop thinking about them until he ate them. He recalled feeling sluggish and ashamed opening a full-size bag then finishing it 30 minutes later. Paul tried to intervene by doing the grocery shopping, yet his partner would inevitably bring them home anyway. Paul begged his partner to not bring them home anymore because they were distracting him from getting work done. The food noise, he said, was intolerable.

His spouse agreed, yet a sort of switch flipped for Paul. Instead of going back to his lunch salads, Paul started to sneak-eat chips during a quick break or on the way home from work. He said he felt like a "junkie" because he felt too ashamed to bring the chips home and eat them in front of his partner.

This sneaking around for potato chips went on for a few years, until Paul's office decided to do a January healthy eating challenge. They picked a popular one demonizing sugary and salty processed foods where certain foods were off limits, including potato chips.

Just like when his mom did a big sweep through his house, Paul's law firm was buzzing with new food rules. Paul was ecstatic when his spouse agreed to do the challenge, too, because then everyone was on board. Paul quickly remembered his role as the healthy office eater and beamed with pride letting me know he lost the most weight in the office. A new switch occurred and he felt empowered enough to no longer drive to the store to sneak-eat chips.

Around this same time, Paul learned about the concept of food addiction and finally had a way to understand his weakness: he could not have the food around because he could not control himself. He was now back to the weight he had maintained while at law school.

I asked Paul why he was coming to meet with me then—it sounded like he had his eating patterns divided up in a way that pleased him.

Paul admitted to me that Gene thought he had food issues. Ever since the healthy eating challenge, Paul only let certain foods in the house and scolded Gene whenever she ate something not allowed. To make matters worse, Paul started to take forever to pick a meal at a restaurant and even avoided family get-togethers with Gene's family because they "didn't eat healthy." Gene said his *healthy eating issues* were getting in the way of Paul actually living a *healthy life*.

Paul said he tried to be more flexible, yet he felt consumed by his thoughts about food. He felt like such a loser because he could take on big cases at work yet not win his "war with his body and mind." Gene shared with him some episodes of my podcast introducing intuitive eating. While loving the concept, Paul said there was no way he could rely on his cravings to dictate his eating choices because he would only eat potato chips and chocolate chip cookies. He had proof: every time he tried to quit dieting he felt out of control.

Paul wasn't a loser. His "out of control" behaviors were predictable. If you, too, relate to the term food addiction or have ever felt out of control with your eating, you are probably experiencing something called *food preoccupation.*

As evolved creatures, we humans have been hardwired to seek food to stay alive. When we get access to enough food consistently and have permission to eat variety, the brain will only think about food when needing to make food decisions. Instead of all the time, a consistently fed brain with permission to eat enough will only think of food when:

- hungry
- connecting with others via food
- making a grocery list
- preparing food.

On the flip side, when enough food is not around, we will fixate on finding another food choice. It will take over the brain as though the food rules have taken it hostage. Picture Ed, that sweaty gym coach, blowing his whistle inside the brain constantly demanding control.

Can you get away from this? Yes, and the steps you take may vary from others, but it won't include eating less. I will share how Paul is mending his history with food in a later chapter. Will he still hold on to the label of food addict? Will you? Only time will tell.

Distraction #5: Diets disguise their connection to white supremacy

I was a big ball of anxiety waiting for my phone to ring. I left a message with a potential dietetic internship preceptor at a big area hospital. I remember pacing while holding the phone in my hand.

My friend laughed at my visible nerves and said, "Why are you nervous? You already got an internship." She had a point, but landing a hospital placement was my next step in the overwhelming laundry list of requirements to become a registered dietitian. I felt unprepared for all the steps, and I had this looming dread that someone was going to find out I did not actually meet the requirements to be a dietitian. I didn't tell my friend that I had recurring nightmares of being found out for skipping a college class and being sent back to finish my degree instead of starting this internship.

My friend piped up, "Oh that's just imposter syndrome, silly!" I had never heard of this term, and since this was pre-Google, I relied on my friend's answer.

Pauline Clance and Dr. Suzanne Imes started using the phrase *imposter syndrome* in their 1978 article "The imposter phenomenon in high achieving women: dynamics and therapeutic intervention."[10] I learned that, when I felt like a fraud, this was imposter syndrome. When I heard about the source of my misguided anxiety, I relaxed for a moment, only to jump again when the phone rang.

I heard hospital background noises as the preceptor set up the time and date for my interview. She told me to meet her in a busy main lobby. Because this was before cell phones, I wondered aloud how the preceptor would know it was me. She stated, "Oh, all dietitians look alike. I am sure I will know when I see you."

I remember breathing a big sigh of relief when I hung up the phone.

At the time, I wondered if that relief came from learning about imposter syndrome. Maybe naming it had helped me relax? It didn't quite match up, yet I moved on to the next thing on my overwhelming to-do list. I felt a similar calmness when that preceptor did recognize me in the lobby. I felt special and as though I belonged. Maybe I'm not a fraud after all because this dietitian thinks I look like one already?

Twenty years later I sat on a tense Zoom call with probably hundreds of dietitians learning from Black colleagues about the deep-rooted racism within dietetics. Mention of the costly dietetic internship as a big barrier brought me back to that busy hospital lobby where I met the preceptor.

That relief, I realized, wasn't from naming imposter syndrome or because I had been recognized. I belonged in that moment because I benefited from white supremacy.

We dietitians spend years studying the human body in privileged academic institutions. The coveted dietetic internship required most of us to move hundreds of miles away from our home without financial aid and needing a car. Outside employment was impossible because of the heavy workload.

It's easy to see the overwhelming whiteness within dietetics since 91 percent of dietitians are white.[11] What was not easy for me to see and is still painful now is how diets were invented to protect whiteness.

Black dietitians finally given the floor to speak during the 2020 United States' racial reckoning spelled out for me the racial origins of diets and diet industry. Dietitians make decisions on how to teach healthy eating, decide worldwide nutrition policy and guidelines, and train the next generation of dietitians. With most dietitians being white and financially secure, it's easy to connect how nutrition education just teaches folks how to eat like a thin, financially stable white person.

How do dietitians define healthy eating?

I learned healthy eating through the lens of the 1992 Food Guide Pyramid. Every dietitian carried copies of it in tear-off sheets to hand out, whether at the hospital or community clinic, showing people how to eat more foods from the bottom and less from the top. I can still see the carbohydrate-rich foods illustrated in the pyramids, showing us good choices that included bread, pasta, crackers, and cereals. I knew these foods because I grew up with them at every meal. The only food not Eurocentric—white rice—would be excluded later when we were told to recommend only brown rice. But what about tortillas, naan, or injera? Why didn't the graphic include anything else outside of white culture?

Fruits and vegetables sat right above and included pictures of these food items in their raw, unprocessed form. We saw produce only available in grocery stores and choices not typically represented in Black, Indigenous, or people of color's homes. Corn, a staple in Hispanic and Latin cultures, had zero representation on this food permission slip.

As a dietitian, I frequently asked people how they prepared their fruits and vegetables, so I could catch the hidden sources of disease-promoting ingredients and reeducate them on "better" ways of eating. I was taught to discourage collard greens, a common vegetable in Black foodways where I live in the southern US, because it was often cooked with fatback. Fatback was a necessary part of the recipe: it provided collard greens their flavor and helped the absorption of the many nutrients in collard greens, such as vitamins A and C, calcium, vitamins K and B_6, and magnesium.

Moving up the pyramid, we saw even more Eurocentric foodways promoting milk and dairy products as well as proteins like meat, eggs, fish, and beans. The tip represented what was to be used only sparingly. This included fats, oils, and sweets, and, to many dietitians, non-Eurocentric ways of preparing foods like collard greens.

Throughout the 1990s and early 2000s, we dietitians famously "healthified" recipes to remove sugar and fat without considering its impact on cultural food connections. As Atkins, Sugar Busters!, and other low-carb diets increased in popularity, I needed to add more fiber to these recommendations. White rice was no longer "healthy," and I could only recommend brown rice. Even though it only provided one more gram of fiber per serving, brown rice significantly impacted taste and texture. I was never trained to appreciate how important that was to an individual eating white rice with every meal as every generation had before them.

The Food Guide Pyramid lost its popularity because of its heavy carbohydrate recommendations, and, in 2011, dietitians were encouraged to move to MyPlate. This placed more emphasis on the type of carbohydrate, pushing fiber and whole grains. Fruits and vegetables were now supposed to be half the food we eat. Frozen and canned were named as options instead of just fresh produce— great news for those relying on shelf-stable options (yet not for long). Sadly, only Eurocentric food staples were listed as examples and thus considered the best choices.

The Mediterranean diet

Current healthy eating trends include minimally processed plant-based foods and vegetable oils. US physiologist Ancel Keys first described this favored eating pattern as the *Mediterranean diet*, based on cultural foods of Greece and Southern Italy.[12]

The *Dietary Guidelines for Americans, 2020–2025* encourages people to mimic this region's eating habits by further increasing fruits, vegetables, fish, and olive oil and heavily restricting red meats, high-fat dairy, saturated fats, and sugars. While this represents part of the Mediterranean region's diaspora, it excludes Eastern European, Middle Eastern, and North African countries. Why are the Mediterranean regions that include Black, Brown, and other people of color excluded?

The guidelines mention including foods you prefer, cultural traditions, and what is accessible. Unfortunately, they override attempts to include different perspectives outside of white culture by cautioning us throughout to be careful. The tag line is: "The Dietary Guidelines for Americans provide science-based advice to help everyone—no matter their age, race, socioeconomic, or health status—achieve better health by *making every bite count*" (emphasis mine). Throughout the document itself, teaching guides, and consumer tear sheets, we are told that Americans don't know how to eat healthily, and we weigh too much, but they neglect to mention we are living longer, too. Of note, while we see folks of different ethnicities and races represented in the infographics, all bodies are thin.

Close your eyes. Imagine a plate of food that we would call healthy. What is on it? Most people have told me some variation of this:

- plain baked salmon
- kale with another colorful vegetable tossed in olive oil
- quinoa or baked sweet potato.

Next, imagine the type of store where this type of food came from. Did you picture some grocery store in a mostly white, affluent neighborhood? This food could not be purchased in American neighborhoods experiencing a lack of food markets, ones relying on food purchases from gas stations and discount stores.

The role of oppressive systems

As dietitians continue to promote healthy food, the diet industry takes these cues and runs with them. Corporations know if a dietitian labels a food "healthy," they will increase their sales with this marketing tactic, so now the foods recommended within the Greek and Southern Italian foodways are *healthy* and *good*, with the rest *bad*. With this signifier, they can also drastically increase the price for consumers.

As the diet industry increases its influence, folks already in power because of race, class, and wealth gain more power by eating the correct combination of foods. These same folks believe they are controlling their health through individual food choices. If they are lowering their A1C level and blood pressure by having a kale salad at lunch every day, then those with chronic health conditions like diabetes must be just too lazy or incompetent to improve their health. Or, they just don't want to be healthy.

Blaming an individual is easier than oppressive systems because it maintains the status quo. Dietitians and the *Dietary Guidelines for Americans* have convinced us we are choosing the wrong foods making us unhealthy. This uplifted the diet industry to control what we should and should not eat. What if, instead, we center the research on social determinants of health and its impact on health and mortality? You and I both know there's no amount of kale you can eat to combat the negative health effects of racism, poverty, and other oppressive systems.

The diet industry uplifts and centers racist beliefs. It has convinced us that:

- white people food is the only healthy food
- cultural foods not associated with Eurocentric traditions cause chronic disease or leave you vulnerable to developing chronic diseases
- the diet industry's food recommendations will give us access to health and vitality
- healthy eating is white rich people food that only rich people can afford.[13]

How do dietitians define healthy weight?

I learned about the Body Mass Index (BMI) in one of my first nutrition undergraduate classes. Using a formula including height and weight, it claimed to determine someone's health risk. But my professors said it did not take into account age, race, or ethnicity, or give us any real insight into muscle mass or body fat percentage. We were advised to use it as just one piece of information.

Years later, the healthcare and diet industries plastered green, yellow, and red BMI charts anywhere with enough wall space. Another tear-off sheet to hand to patients to jolt them into behavior change if they fell into the red high-BMI zone. Most of us know by now that we need a BMI of 18.5–24.9 to be deemed healthy—but why? How did this number—which really doesn't give us that much information—get this power over us?

BMI was not invented by a dietitian or doctor. Belgian Adolphe Quetelet wasn't even in healthcare. In 1832, Quetelet sought out a way to quantify the characteristics of a "normal man" and used his skills as a statistician, mathematician, and astronomer to come up with the calculator we use today. Ancel Keys used this formula to analyze a 7000-plus population of "healthy" men. Keys came up with the name Body Mass Index and noted it was a convenient tool to analyze *data*... not necessarily individuals.[14]

What is a "normal" person? How did researchers decide who was a "healthy" person?

Diverse shapes, including plump physiques common in Renaissance art, were considered healthy throughout world history until the 17th century.

According to sociologist Dr. Sabrina Strings, this changed as European men started to characterize fatness as displeasing. With the transatlantic slave trade booming, Europeans desired to distinguish and categorize all sorts of new and diverse people from most desirable to least desirable. The slave trade violently dehumanized Black Africans, and Europeans judged their traumatized human reaction to this violence as evidence of white superiority. Darker skin and rounder bodies became code for inferiority and lack of intelligence. The Protestant religion enhanced this code and added an immoral dimension to fatness.[15]

Uniquely American at first, white thinness became en vogue in the early 19th century. Blackness equated savagery whereas whiteness meant discipline. The thinner one became, the more distinctly not Black one was regarded. This elevated a thin person's place in society, opened up opportunities within academia and employment, and, especially for women, helped them marry. Anti-fat bias began in the US among the morally elite, and thinness and whiteness became the sign of American exceptionalism.[16]

Before the BMI took off, the insurance companies found those outside of average weight-to-height ratios were at highest mortality risk. Of course, they used data from their policyholders, aka working-age, middle-class, salaried employed white men. Normal and healthy weight ideals excluded everyone else. Insurance companies eventually developed the widely used Metropolitan Life Tables, which like BMI, determined everyone's health using only white subjects. Normal and healthy weight was determined (and still is) mostly by white, middle-aged men.

Because thinness equated morality, intellect, class, and good health, industries invented tools and methods for consumers. This became the diet industry, rooting for you and me to stay thin while they rake in over $70 billion in the US yearly. I was taught a healthy weight prolonged health but not the history of *how* we came to this information. Without regarding our intergenerational history on weight attitudes, it is easy to miss how as a dietitian I was trained to help someone distinguish themselves from Blackness. I was trained to code healthy weight as a more superior white elite.

If the history of weight science is new to you, please do not stop here. I encourage you to next learn from those most impacted by anti-fatness. I have listed places to begin in the Resources section of this book.

Dietitians are diet industry's line leaders enthusiastically chanting the battle cry that individuals can and should control their weight. Those unable or unwilling are cast aside and shamed, losing proximity to thinness and thus whiteness.

Many of my clients have wondered why diets are so painful to stop doing. You, too, may have contemplated this after decades of diets not working for you. Here's the secret you now know: the diet industry has immoral, violent beginnings in racism. This secret origin laid the foundation for your *I-Should-Eat* scripts. It was downloaded into your brain without your consent, dictating a set of instructions to elevate you. For some this script was a means to higher status whereas for others it provided vital safety. While painful, hold this while contemplating food choices moving forward. We were not told the truth about dieting's origins, yet now we can do better.

Distraction #6: Diets disguise their connection to the patriarchy and capitalism

I still remember how I felt after watching the viral "Shrinking Women" poem written and performed by Lily Myers.[17] Probably sleep-deprived giving my infant son a bottle at 5 a.m., I felt rage, desperation, and joy listening to her slam poetry describing her experiences as a cisgender woman in her family and her observed jealous dichotomy compared to men in her life.

Within just three minutes, Myers conveys how women are taught to restrict food yet are gaslit to believe they have plenty.

Myers describes her mom's obvious self-denial at meal time focusing on how little to eat. Even though her mom tries to cover up these acts, Myers appreciates how her mom's behavior is teaching to deny food pleasure as a default setting and only eat when told it's time to eat.

She compares her mom's situation with her dad's. She describes him as proudly expanding with new ideas and abundant self-permission to weigh more. His girlfriend, though, has learned how to limit her pleasure with food by lying to herself about healthy food preferences.

When did we learn men should always eat more than women? Listening to Myers recite this poem captivated me even in my sleep-deprived haze because she showed me how starkly differently men and women are raised. She shows how obvious it is, yet somehow we are all under the same spell.

One thing I know as a dietitian: not eating enough is exhausting. What's even more tiring? Planning family meals, grocery shopping, and food prep while not eating enough. A brain requires more energy than any other organ and not eating enough will make thoughts spacey, distracted, and forgetful.

Why do we succumb to to diets? Are we just obsessed with looking pretty? No. It goes so much deeper. Naomi Wolf, author of the *Beauty Myth*, teaches how it's not about being pretty. It's about using the concept of beauty and all that goes into making one look a specific way is a rather sly way to control and keep a population quiet about what is actually wrong.[18] Wolf is saying: dieting will make your brain unable to fight back and see what industries are doing to keep you stuck. It's tough to see how oppressive systems complicate your food history or your life in general. As I mentioned while discussing food preoccupation, not eating enough will make your brain prioritize food thoughts over everything else.

Myers emphasizes this in "Shrinking Women": she describes asking questions in genetics class all starting with an apology—her words figuratively trying to be careful. Later Myers reports missing out on key information about degree requirements because her brain debated on whether or not to eat another piece of pizza.

A consequence of racism is sexism—the power structures giving cisgender men more societal power. The diet industry has found a place first in women's food history to keep us fixated on staying relevant and pleasing to the male gaze. We women were gaslit to believe that we have no control over food, yet controlling it to stay thin is the only way to stay seen by men. We've been manipulated to prioritize that male gaze so much that we don't even see it anymore. It has become that fundamental. At its core, diet control helps us do the dirty work of uplifting cisgender white men to maintain power.

I raged watching Myers's poetry that dark early morning. I watched that performance so many times I could recite the entire poem later that day. If you were sitting on my green therapy room couch that day, you were in the direct line of my feminist fire. A three-minute YouTube video summed up my feminist anti-diet belief system (regretfully still lacking much intersection with other systems of oppression mostly because sexism was the only one I faced).

Over the years, I am grateful to the work of authors Dr. Sabrina Strings and Da'Shaun L. Harrison who have helped me to appreciate how sexism is not the foundation rather just a system rooted in racism.

Specializing in PCOS, I witnessed patriarchal control disguised in overly simplified diet recommendations. As I read through Matilda's tear-stained food journal years ago, I asked her what she knew about PCOS. She was surprised there was anything to know. I was surprised by her surprise! PCOS impacts just about every cell in the body. Matilda recounted her simple instructions when diagnosed: "Here's birth control, focus on weight loss, and come back when you are trying to get pregnant."

Because of sexism, like most people with PCOS, Matilda was led to believe that she needed to only worry about weight and her ability to reproduce. Healthcare providers minimized PCOS's impact on her quality of life because of the providers' overfocus on the traditional woman's role: stay pretty (read: thin) and carry a pregnancy to term. Focus on attracting that male gaze. Come back for medical support when you are doing your lady duty of creating another worker. Cue my fired-up eye roll. Twenty-year-old me would call this taking it too far, yet now, with my almost fifty years, I am sounding the alarm.

Matilda was led to believe she alone could improve her chronic illness through weight loss, and the only thing needing more intensive medical attention was her reproductive role in this world. When Matilda didn't successfully lose weight, she was told she wasn't trying hard enough. When she complained of fatigue, migraines, mood swings, and other common PCOS symptoms, healthcare providers failed to provide meaningful support outside of pushing diets to fix it. Even worse, doctors told her that it was her lack of willpower and weight gain that caused these PCOS symptoms.

When PCOS affects one in seven women and those born with a uterus, why did Matilda know so little? Is it just a mistake? Is it just too tough to figure out?

Of course not. Sexist systems run PCOS healthcare—it's no secret that most doctors and researchers are white cisgender men.[19] Without lived experience informing care, it's easy to discount PCOS symptoms as just being in a woman's head.

A healthcare system overemphasizing an individual's food and exercise behaviors fits nicely into checking all the boxes on a doctor's to-do list. It also falls in line with current power structures centering white cisgender men and gaslighting the rest of us into believing we just can't do it correctly. The tradition keeps our attention believing we cause our own suffering even when complying with the *I-Should-Eat* script. Taking giant steps back, I hope you are beginning to see the billions of people stuck looking at a set of instructions while a few pour jet fuel on the problems and profit via capitalistic distraction.

Distraction #7: Diets disguise the harm from weight stigma

The diet industry has trained us to believe that we can tell how someone eats just by looking at them. My higher-weight clients have used their size as proof they obviously have to eat less.

Were you bullied as a child because of how you looked? I remember watching friends get harassed at school because of their size. Higher-weight colleagues tell me about how it is hard for them to find jobs. Weight stigma is something that we will often see as bullying at school, harassment, violence, dehumanization, hostility, negative appearance commentary, pressures to lose weight, and many other weight-related microaggressions.

Clients told me they were getting teased at school and that, whenever they would go to a trusted adult to try to stop the bullying, they said, "Let's help you lose weight so they will stop." If we were dealing with anybody else being teased, we would never tell them to change so that people would stop teasing them. We wouldn't tell the victim to fix themselves; we would get the bullies to stop. There's something pervasive about weight and weight bias that keeps that from happening.

Weight stigma dehumanizes higher-weight bodies and happens every day in the media. Have you watched the news and seen people at higher weights shown without their heads visible or their eyes marked out with that black bar? When people at higher weights are not shown in a way that's normal, respectable, and dignified, it makes a person look less like a human. When we dehumanize people, it's one of the steps right before violence. It's much more common for people at higher weights to experience violence, and this dehumanization plays a part.[20]

Only one state in the US (Michigan) has laws against discrimination based on weight and the hiring process. In 49 states, someone could go up to a higher-weight person and say, "You know what, you'd be the perfect person for this job, but you're too fat, so we will not hire you," and it is perfectly legal. This is not okay.

Weight stigma is not always obvious. Sometimes it is subtle. Don't let the smallness sway you from seeing the big impact. Microaggressions are usually unintentional yet still harmful. They can be verbal, behavioral, or even systemic indignities that let people know that they're in a hostile or negative environment just being themselves.

Appearance-based comments seem like a positive yet provide one whip of microaggression. Complimentary weightism sounds like: "You've lost weight, you're looking good." This is stigmatizing because, although positive on the surface, it still marks people out as good or bad based on weight.

Not only does weight-based stigma make people feel more shame, but it is also harmful to their health. Weight stigma is related to hypertension, inflammation, high triglycerides, higher calorie intake, binge eating, other eating disorder behaviors, and depression. So really understanding weight bias and how it affects health is important. Putting all this together, though, gets uncomfortable because it is political.

Weight bias *is* political because it talks about policies, laws, how we treat people, and how people have access to health. This informs how I vote. As I say that, please know that it doesn't necessarily mean you have to be a conservative or liberal to move away from diets. People identify as either one and fight against weight discrimination. Yet, know that it does inform my political views and who I vote for. It may for you, too.

All the distractions that have led you to this

I have a feeling that, if you are in a higher-weight body, then you have gone to the doctor and they assumed you eat way more than you actually do. They may also give you exercise recommendations without even checking to see that you are already doing more than the recommendation.

How frustrating for you!

Weight-loss providers emphasize one should keep trying to lower weight to improve health yet de-emphasize diet failure rate and the costs of weight cycling. In order for a higher-weight individual to be deemed officially healthy, they must practice an eating disorder, though that is no guarantee. Even with restrictions and overexercise, you may still not be small enough for many healthcare providers because weight loss itself is not a behavior.

If you are in a higher-weight body, your size is not the problem! Dieting behaviors are the disease, not your body size.

If you are not in a higher-weight body, these assumptions are drilled into your brain, too, leading to a fear of weight gain and contributing to discrimination against higher-weight people. We all have this because we were brought up within the powerful diet industry, and we must be aware of it to remove it. Not only will that help your higher-weight friends and the higher-weight community, but it will also help you remove the shame and blame you feel for your eating and exercise decisions. Diet industry seductions hurt all of us and only together can we stop them.

Weight loss and food restriction won't fit with the goal of healing your relationship with food. They only enhance that food noise from food preoccupation. As a long-term eating disorder provider, I have learned the way to move away from food preoccupation is through ending your diet cycle. Anyone who complains of binge eating, emotional eating, food noise, or food addiction can only move away from this chaotic existence by no longer dieting. Weight loss will not cure this.

Before the Big Cry, I tried to help people move away from diets and pursue weight loss. In order to heal your relationship with food, it is important to hold on to this new *knowing* that weight cannot be sustainably lowered with food restrictions and overexercise. This takes time to unravel especially because our world will just tangle it up again each day.

So why do you blame yourself when a diet fails?

- If diets don't work for most people, why do doctors and dietitians recommend them?
- If diets are the answer, why do we have to keep going on them?
- If diets are actually harmful long term—promoting weight cycling, higher insulin levels, higher triglycerides, higher blood sugars, depression, and negative body image—why are they recommended to improve health?

Those are important questions with a really nasty answer: The world contains so much anti-fat bias stemming from racism it cannot wrap its head around the notion that weight loss is not a behavior. Medical science has yet to find ONE diet that works to promote health and promote maintenance long-term for most people. The diet industry controls the narrative, convincing us we can control our weight with their tools and keep us stuck in the Diet Trap.

We see how people of size are treated in our world. Chairs don't fit, airplanes won't accommodate, and culture hasn't provided equal treatment in academia, the military, or employment.

This constant weight-based discrimination keeps anyone stuck in the Diet Trap. Every human needs a place to belong and feel safe. Pursuing weight loss, with all its hopeful sparks, holds the promise for ease in a world that says their body is not acceptable.

My higher-weight clients shared that, when dieting, they felt as though at least they were complying with the world's orders, providing a sliver more acceptance and safety.

You have done all that it takes to weigh less, even when it hurt. Each time you complied with the diet orders, the fantasy of equal treatment and a better life filled your head.

This is the *I-Should-Eat* script

Intuitive eating and other non-diet tools may have failed you because of the seductive magnetic pull from your many scripts. You may have an intellectual understanding of these anti-diet concepts, yet they are not working because of how the diet industry keeps pulling you back in. You are just doing what you are told while craving equality and decency.

Unfortunately, the *I-Should-Eat* script distracts us all from the fact that diets don't work for most people and they are harmful. It distracts us from the bigotry that comes from weight stigma, racism, gender inequality, and all the other systems of oppression.

The *I-Should-Eat* script is so close to our faces in every breath we take, it manages to be invisible. Ignorance is bliss for the least marginalized, yet it keeps us from truth. We are rewarded for not naming the diet industry with the thick hopefulness of being seen and heard.

As a thin white person, I could have just kept living my life pretending the script wasn't there. Remember when I cried in my boss's office? In that moment I could no longer unsee these systems of oppression, especially in my nutrition recommendations. I was building *I-Should-Eat* scripts—lying that I had the keys to freedom when in reality I was just another diet industry line leader.

I had started to unpack dieting's connection to racism and my role in uplifting it. I unpacked so much that it no longer could fit inside the toxic positivity I relied on.

It just took a moment for me to hold on to this new-to-me truth to turn my head gently to consider another way to relate to food, body, and movement.

I wonder if you can turn your head slightly now, too? Consider for a moment that you have never failed dieting. You are not doing it wrong. Rather, you are following the rules exactly as they have been written and drank the dripped-out sugar-free Kool-Aid convincing you that you need more diet rules. These rules were downloaded without your consent, promising freedom yet just keeping more tightly chained to feelings of shame and blame. They have kept you stuck in the Diet Trap.

Even while you are still shackled with unworthiness, let's call out the real villain. It's not you; it's all of your *I-Should-Eat* scripts. It's the oppressive systems created out of racism. You are not alone in connecting with all of this. I am with you in solidarity, radically rejecting diets and mending your own innate wisdom for health.

It is time for you to take off that shame cloak. It is not for you. It never was. Taking the cloak off, though, may be like bumping a scab off a painful injury. Instead of just applying another Band-Aid that keeps you holding on to the shame, I invite you to keep going. Where you go next will transform the wounds into repaired armor. You will be stronger, ready to help the stranger behind you find their Food Voice, too.

Dear Kim,

> We are sitting with you in this sadness and grief. Do you notice how brave you are seeing the world for what it is? Naming the evils and power-hungry systems disguised as what saves us? You took the leap, and while this path is a slippery slope, you are contributing to the repair. Keep going. Take breaks when you need it. When you notice the shame, remind yourself of its origins. Stay fueled and awake because we need you in this fight.

> Love,
> Food

Dear Food letter activity

Write a letter to Food describing your Diet Trap and the oppressive systems that brought you there. Name *all* of them. Describe them in as much detail as fits for you. Call them out for their injustice and how that affected your ability to trust yourself and the world.

References

1 *United States Weight Loss and Diet Control Market* (2023). Marketdata Enterprises.
2 Kingsley, L. (2023). The seesawing history of fad diets: since dieting began in the 1830s, the ever-changing nutritional advice has skimped on science. *The Smithsonian Magazine*, February 7. https://www.smithsonianmag. com/innovation/the-seesawing-history-of-fad-diets-180981586/ (accessed April 24, 2024).
3 "White supremacy," *Merriam-Webster Collegiate Dictionary*, https://www. merriam-webster.com/dictionary/white%20supremacy (accessed April 24, 2024).
4 Mann, T., Tomiyama, A. J., Westling, E., Lew, A.-M., Samuels, B., & Chatman, J. (2007). Medicare's search for effective obesity treatments: diets are not

the answer. *American Psychologist* 62(3), 220–33. https://doi.org/10.1037/0003-066x.62.3.220.

5 Hall, K. D., & Kahan, S. (2018). Maintenance of lost weight and long-term management of obesity. *Medical Clinics of North America* 102(1), 183–97. https://doi.org/10.1016/j.mcna.2017.08.012.

6 Mahmood, S. S., Levy, D., Vasan, R. S., & Wang, T. J. (2014). The Framingham Heart Study and the epidemiology of cardiovascular disease: a historical perspective. *The Lancet* 383(9921), 999–1008. https://doi.org/10.1016/s0140-6736(13)61752-3.

7 Rzehak, P., Meisinger, C., Woelke, G., Brasche, S., Strube, G., & Heinrich, J. (2007). Weight change, weight cycling, and mortality in the Erfort Male Cohort Study. *Aktuelle Ernährungsmedizin* 32(05). https://doi.org/10.1055/s-2007-992295.

8 Field, A. E., Manson, J. E., Taylor, C. B., Willett, W. C., & Colditz, G. A. (2004). Association of weight change, weight control practices, and weight cycling among women in the Nurses' Health Study II. *International Journal of Obesity* 28(9), 1134–42.

9 Fothergill, E., Guo, J., Howard, L., Kerns, J. C., Knuth, N. D., Brychta, R., Chen, K. Y., Skarulis, M. C., Walter, M., Walter, P. J., & Hall, K. D. (2016). Persistent metabolic adaptation 6 years after "The Biggest Loser" competition. *Obesity* (Silver Spring, MD) 24(8), 1612–19. https://doi.org/10.1002/oby.21538.

10 Clance, P., & Imes, S. (1978). The imposter phenomenon in high achieving women: dynamics and therapeutic intervention. *Psychotherapy: Theory, Research & Practice* 15(3), 241–7.

11 https://www.diversifydietetics.org/blog-1/2018/4/24/its-time-to-change-the-face-of-nutrition (accessed September 21, 2023).

12 Davis, C., Bryan, J., Hodgson, J., & Murphy, K. (2015). Definition of the Mediterranean diet: a literature review. *Nutrients* 7(11), 9139–53. https://doi.org/10.3390/nu7115459.

13 https://www.healthline.com/health/nutrition/who-gets-to-be-healthy#18 (accessed May 20, 2024); https://www.thefoodhistorian.com/blog/are-nutrition-science-and-nutritional-guidelines-racist (accessed May 20, 2024).

14 Pray, R., & Riskin, S. (2023). The history and faults of the body mass index and where to look next: a literature review. *Cureus* 15(11). https://doi.org/10.7759/cureus.48230.

15 Strings, S. (2019). *Fearing the Black Body: The Racial Origins of Fat Phobia*. New York University Press.

16 Ibid.

17 https://www.youtube.com/watch?v=02DDpoZ-Kg8 (accessed October 2, 2023).

18 Wolf, N. (1990). *The Beauty Myth: How Images of Beauty Are Used Against Women*. Chatto & Windus.

19 https://www.statista.com/statistics/439731/share-of-physicians-by-specialty-and-gender-in-the-us/ (accessed April 24, 2024).

20 Kersbergen, I., & Robinson, E. (2019). Blatant dehumanization of people with obesity. *Obesity* 27(6), 1005–12. https://doi.org/10.1002/oby.22460.

3

Definition

Dear Food,

Ever since I can remember, I was an insecure child who struggled with her body image. I wasn't even a heavy child, just so embarrassed about my body. Additionally, I was exposed to diet culture early on as the women in my family, especially my mother, had become so invested in the restrictions of a diet that it was all they could talk about, ultimately crashing and burning later on. I adopted the idea that the Atkins Diet was the cure; it had to be with the way my family sang its praises... even though it really never changed the way they looked.

In high school, I struggled with a binging and purging disorder. No, actually, I still wrestle with those thoughts all the time, and every now and again I give in, which in the moment feels like a terrible itch I'm finally getting to scratch. Food is comfort for me. It doesn't matter if I'm stressed, tired, or happy ... I want to eat! I love to eat, and large amounts in a single sitting, too, though I prefer the meal to be of quality ingredients and not something like fast food. Not that my relationship with food is of much quality in itself.

Fast-forward to 2018. I was being given some concerning news about an abnormal pap smear and the doctor wanted to perform a procedure to help eliminate these bad cells ... Only I wasn't having it. I decided I wanted to follow a keto diet and heal myself naturally. Well ... it actually worked. And even better, I lost 25 pounds while doing it. Over time, I started slacking, eventually gaining it all back. Since then, I've been chasing the dream that I could lose those 25 pounds on the keto diet again, but it's just not the same. I have very little success, especially with the pandemic changing so many physical requirements I once had. I still try, still cheat, still try again … try to change my focus to healthy eating like in the old days, but I have lost sight of what that was. Was it the giant salads for lunch? Or those bone broth–only lunches? Was it macro tracking, or the ten-plus different supplements I took every day? Who knows now?

I'm now 16 weeks postpartum, delivered via C-section. My confidence is shot. I try to appear like it's not, but my partner can see right through me. I'm also breastfeeding and have already decreased my milk supply once, so anything else makes me terrified. My remedy for that is just to eat whatever I want whenever I want, and that's not good.

I just want to be in control of myself when it comes to using food for comfort. I'm so tired of thinking about diets, it's exhausting. I want a snack just thinking about it, and I wish it was a joke, but it isn't.

From Kayla

What the hell is intuitive eating anyway, and why is it everywhere?

I was about ready to quit dietetics in 2002. That year, I took a leave of absence from my hospital dietitian job and started graduate school in mental health counseling. As I trained the dietitian, Alice, who would be taking over my responsibilities on my last day, I admitted to her I wouldn't be a dietitian much longer. Curious, Alice asked me why. I told her I just didn't think diets worked and what a person ate had so little to do with their worth.

Alice suggested I read one book before quitting: *Intuitive Eating*.

Thank you, Alice, for suggesting this because it did indeed keep me from quitting dietetics. I have mentioned this book because it likely has come across your radar already. Evelyn Tribole and Elyse Resch first wrote the book *Intuitive Eating* in 1995, and it brought a concrete consumer option to a diet-obsessed 1990s and 2000s. It wasn't the first non-diet book yet it was the one that started measuring outcomes to catch healthcare providers' attention. It certainly caught mine and greatly impacted my understanding of our Food Voice.

Intuitive eating's core message states that *we all have unconditional permission to eat—no matter our size*. In order to repair a complicated history with food, working toward unconditional permission will lead to a more neutral experience.

As intuitive eating gained traction with the advent of Twitter and Instagram, I noticed most of the chatter around it lacked this concept of permission. Most intuitive eating conversations centered on the hunger/fullness scale. Using a line graph numbered 1 through 10, Tribole and Resch describe the process of getting to know the physical sensations of hunger (with 1 being very hungry) versus the physical sensations of fullness (with 10 being uncomfortably full).

Using your physical body cues can be a useful tool to repair your relationship with food, but it is not the only way. Even more, some folks I have met do not share the same interoceptive connections. Others find hunger and fullness conversations inaccessible or not helpful. If we center hunger as permission to eat, what about folks experiencing food insecurity? Famine?

Finding *your* Food Voice may or may not include noticing hunger and fullness. It is not a requirement. Further, I find too many people build hunger and fullness scales with the same rigid diet mentality that eventually permission to eat is only granted with hunger.

This is not your Food Voice. This is not permission. This is a one-way ticket back to your Diet Trap.

I encourage you to de-center hunger as the be-all and end-all way to approve putting food into your mouth. Instead, concentrate on increasing your permission to eat even outside of hunger. Give yourself permission to soothe, comfort, and celebrate with food. It is okay if this feels especially wrong or immoral. You are literally firing up your scripts to react. I will teach you in Chapter 5 how to set up guardrails to move away from these triggered scripts.

Will I ever feel normal around food?

Just like this chapter's letter writer, most folks I know struggle with realistically picturing a normal relationship with food. People have told me about their out-of-reach dreams of eating a relaxed lunch with friends or having a midday snack without counting macros. This feels like a fantasy because of the outside pressure to look a certain way as well as the ever-present bad body thoughts. Making the big moves away from dieting probably feels impossible. I remember Matilda, one of my first clients with PCOS, saying she just didn't feel strong enough to leave off diets as a way of managing her eating. Most people on her college campus were thin, and as one of the few higher-weight students, not dieting was not an option in Matilda's mind.

The book *Intuitive Eating* became more popular in the early 2000s and 2010s, so I was hopeful that anti-diet ways of eating would be welcomed and normalized on college campuses. I hoped Matilda wouldn't be radical, allowing her to reject weight loss goals and manage her health on her own terms. I hoped people would see the diet industry for what it was: a complex disguised delusion distracting us from oppressive systems.

While more people entertained the idea of not dieting, folks like Matilda tried to give up dieting yet still felt overloaded with constant food and body worries. *Intuitive Eating* appeared to help for a little while yet the food noise got too loud and clients reported feeling like a failure again. Many felt even more burdened with intuitive eating because eating felt more chaotic. It was like someone took a dial and turned up the food noise.

Failing tools like intuitive eating may have felt even harder for you because it was supposed to be *the* way out.

If this sounds like your experience, please know you didn't do intuitive eating wrongly. Somehow along the way, diet companies learned about intuitive eating's popularity and swiftly changed their marketing messages. They learned new non-dieting words to just blanket on top of their diets as they tried to fool us. Be wary of the diet industry's shapeshifting vocabulary that combines intuitive eating buzzwords with diet concepts and slogans:

- Mindful eating to eat less
- Healthy eating without dieting
- Body-positive weight loss
- Change your mindset
- There are no bad foods just bad portions

- Stop emotionally eating and only eat when hungry
- It's not a diet! (Don't trust them on it!).

At the same time, applying intuitive eating principles in a dieting world got lost in translation, making food choices more complicated. I noticed clients applying intuitive eating principles just as they would a diet. Intuitive eating became the "intuitive eating diet"—only eating when hungry and stopping when full.

If you feel like you failed at intuitive eating, know you didn't do it wrongly. You are just missing a tool to reconnect with your own innate wisdom to eat, as discussed in *Intuitive Eating*.

I want to help you reconnect with that wisdom. I wrote this chapter to help you start that reconnection that will only get stronger over time. While this chapter will get you started, you will find your Food Voice one *aha!*, one conversation, one courageous act at a time.

The complexity of your Food Voice

I don't think anyone currently exists who is purely aligned with just their Food Voice—and yes, that includes me. Let's set expectations: while reconnecting to your own innate way of eating without diets, do not expect perfection. Do not expect to always follow a new way of eating, rigidly giving yourself permission to eat only when certain circumstances line up. This is how intuitive eating gets twisted back into a diet, and the same goes with finding your Food Voice. As a newly minted Voice Finder, grant yourself permission to make mistakes, get messy, and not always move forward. Remember, you are getting out of that rental car garage with the spikes. It may feel easier in the moment to always go in one direction (following a diet), yet that has kept you in your Diet Trap. Reconnecting with your Food Voice and practicing using it as your guide to food decisions will feel like you are aimlessly drifting sometimes, but that doesn't mean you are going in the wrong direction.

Your Food Voice is innate, yet intergenerational body discrimination has been nestled alongside it. As an infant, you instinctively knew when you needed fuel and comfort as well as when you were satisfied. Unfortunately, your caregivers were breathing in the air full of anti-fat bias and body distrust and were already questioning your hungry baby screams. Your ancestors before you preprogrammed your DNA to be wary of trusting food's pleasure to keep you safe and alive.

To know your Food Voice is to also know what is working against it. Most of this book helps you discern the individual and systemic influences covering up access to your Food Voice so you can weave it—your Food Voice—back together into its own reliable constant, no matter the noise around you.

And there is always noise.

I hope you are ready to meet it differently than you have before.

Your Food Voice is as basic as a tiny cell needing glucose that leads to the complex notification to the rest of your body through hundreds of precise hormonal shifts letting you know it is time to eat. Your Food Voice is as boring as making a grocery list. It is as exciting as biting into a kielbasa connecting to every Polish funeral and wedding you (I) attended. Your Food Voice floods with childhood memories of noshing on that first or tenth Christmastime Buckeye dessert (a peanut butter and chocolate masterpiece from my home state of Ohio), still hours from any hunger cue.

Your Food Voice is primal and complex. It is concrete and multifunctional. Eating food is one of the five core necessities of human existence (along with water, shelter, oxygen, and sleep), yet, depending on where you live and how much access you have, only a reliable option for the privileged.

It's time to reintroduce you to your Food Voice. To begin, here's your magic wand.

Why a magic wand?

Like I mentioned, your Food Voice has always coincided with the diet industry and all of its oppressive systems. I want you to know your Food Voice without the added bullshit. I know uncovering your Food Voice outside of the pressure to diet will help you feel less burdened with your food decisions because it will help you trust yourself again. Unfortunately, the added bullshit has always been there. Each layer of bull comes from years of living within the diet industry and oppressive systems on your unique path. Discerning between what you want to trust and what is ready to turn against you will be tricky and takes a bit of magic.

Another important note: this magic wand needs to be here because your Food Voice is different from mine. In order to repair your food history, you need to access your unique Food Voice. This is your work to do. I don't want to pretend we have the same lived experiences and identities. I want you to connect with your innate language on how to eat, manage food, and all that comes with it. I need to step aside as you make this reconnection.

With this magic wand, I hope it helps you to connect at least for moments at a time with your authentic Food Voice so both of you can reconnect and get to know each other. As you become more familiar with your Food Voice, I will teach you in upcoming chapters how to mend its wounds and how to tend to their repair.

Preparing for your Food Voice

Let's go through a series of questions to help you discern life without the need to diet and without the need to make your body different and/ or perfect. I have adapted this from a guided imagery activity I read in the book *When Women Stop Hating Their Bodies*.[1]

I encourage you to read this next section in a quiet place where you can let your brain roam and you can take your time. While this is my ask, do the best you can with that! If you are holding this book while feeding your baby or vacuuming the living room or some other task, so be it. Just like everything else within this book, there is no best way. You just do what is *your* accessible next step.

Meeting your magic wand

Imagine in this moment seeing a magic wand at your feet. With one glance it is special. You notice its intricate carvings from top to bottom. Someone spent hours making this just for you. Picking it up, you feel how it holds a new energy. It is refreshingly cool to the touch. It has a heaviness that is not a burden, just powerful.

What does it look like? Feel like? Let your brain think through all the descriptions it can. Write them down for future reference. Try to take many mental pictures of your magic wand because we will use them again.

You instinctively wave it—as one does with a magic wand!

And with that wave, instantly there is a difference. You know this wand has been waiting for you to wave it like you did to show its magic.

By waving the wand, you see all the sparkles and glitter float around you. As they swirl, part of the magic also washes around every human on this planet.

All at once, you know everything has changed, yet nothing on the surface appears different.

This magic wand has erased the belief that certain bodies are better than others. The white, cisgender, thin, able body is no longer the ideal, rather it just *is* alongside all the rest of the world's bodies.

While this may sound bananas, stay with me.

Hold this new belief: you and the rest of the planet no longer value thinness and any of its other shrouded synonyms such as muscular, healthy looking, fit, petite, or slim.

All forms of body diversity—age, race, ethnicity, height, weight, ability, and everything not named—exist equally without different privileges.

After waving the magic wand you take all this new knowing in. While your body doesn't change, the way you relate to it does in an instant.

Scan your hands and heart

Look at your hands holding on to the wand and notice every textured inch of skin, hair, veins, moles, and signs of aging. You notice these instead of judging them as flaws. Instead of your usual hypercritical messages, your brain reacts differently.

How does your brain respond to your hands? Now that you and no one else on the planet knows how to negatively judge your body or anyone else's, what do you think?

How do you feel about your hands?

Let yourself look at your hands with this new *knowing*. Wiggle your hands around if you can. Let your thoughts and feelings flow. Give yourself a minute or two and connect with the messages entering your stream of consciousness. If words float into your brain with this new connection, jot them down in a notebook or go to FindYourFoodVoiceBook.com or library. johnmurraylearning.com for a special worksheet for this activity.

After spending as much time as you need and can with your hands, move them to your heart. Find where you can feel it beating. Notice the rhythm it makes and where you can feel it. How long has it been doing this? Moving with this rhythm? An awareness helps you to feel the rhythm and all the other body processes happening all throughout your body without your control.

The glittery spray has barely settled from you waving that powerful stick as you connect with a new sense of gratitude. Where shame for your self-perceived flaws lived, appreciation now fills you up. What color is shame to you? Notice it leaving your body through your feet to the earth. What color is your gratitude? Notice it flowing effortlessly through the top of your head and spreading throughout your body.

What messages do you get if any about this body gratitude? What do you feel? What does your brain appreciate now about your body parts? Give yourself as long as you need and connect with the messages. If words float into your brain with this new connection, jot them down for your future self.

Consider how you would answer these following questions:

- While holding on to this body gratitude, how do you choose what clothes to wear?
- While holding on to this body gratitude, how do you decide what to place in your grocery cart?
- While holding on to this body gratitude, how do you experience your body waiting to be seen by a doctor?
- While holding on to this body gratitude, how do you choose where to sit on the bus?

Food's function is no longer manipulation

The magic wand has brought another new revelation worldwide: eating is a tool for living and connecting. Food brings fuel as well as depth to each moment. How that richness is defined is based on your heritage, culture, preferences, and access.

With the magic wand's powers, food no longer is a tool for body manipulation or power. It just doesn't work that way now. Bodies change with aging, yet food no longer has the power to change body size. As far-fetched as this seems in our current reality, I encourage you to fantasize about this possibility.

No matter how much or little you eat, your body will do what it is genetically programmed to do. Just with the rhythm of your heart, your body systems decide how to use each bite without you needing to worry about it. You know your body will use food in the way it needs. In this new system, that *knowing* is not good or bad—it just is.

Holding these new truths, consider these important questions. Stay with each one as long as you need to let all of your unique messages come through.

With this *knowing*, how do you decide...

- when to eat?
- when to stop eating?
- what food to bring into your home?
- how much food to put on your plate?
- to order food at a restaurant knowing that everyone has also been affected the same way by the magic wand?
- what to put in your grocery cart?
- what snacks to order at the movies?

What about the *shoulds*?

Rae, my client who started dieting in kindergarten, giggled as I took them through the same magic wand guided imagery you just read. I loved seeing them grab the imaginary magic wand and wave it with big circles for effect. I remembered Rae sitting still on my therapy room's green couch and dutifully observing their hands. They took their time looking at the front then back then back to the front again. When they placed their hands over their heart, I noticed tears streaming down Rae's face.

When the guided imagery was over, Rae read the words they had jotted down about their hands in their crisp, new journal: strong, smooth on palm, rough on outside, hairy knuckles, different-length nails, and veins raised up looking like Grandma's hands.

When I gently asked about the tears, Rae shared how long it had been since they felt somewhat neutral about their body. Feeling the pounding of their heart, pulsing with a rhythm going on whether Rae loved or hated their earth suit, they said they felt taken care of in a way they had never felt before. It was a fleeting moment yet it was there and captured.

Finding your Food Voice is hard work and takes time. Capturing that brief moment was a seed of hope for Rae. Over the next few months, we often went back to the actions of observing the hands and having

Rae put them on their heart to help them reunite with hope. Catch your fleeting moments, too! Look for them as they will be the pillars when the *shoulds* creep in.

Just seconds after those grateful tears, Rae let me in on some self-talk. When I asked, "How do you decide when to eat?" they instinctively wrote "When it is time to eat." A few moments later, more details were noted: "Using hunger to help to know when it is time to eat or if friends were gathered to eat a meal. But if not really hungry physically then nothing should be eaten."

I remembered asking: "Are you *shoulding*?"

At this point in our work together, Rae already knew about my cheeky phrase "Stop shoulding on yourself." I learned it back in my counseling training as a way to detect shame with gentle humor.

Shame never promotes repair with your eating history. It also doesn't promote health (much to the chagrin of most healthcare providers).

Making decisions on when to eat and how much to eat quickly moved to a dieting lens for Rae. It may for you, too. This doesn't mean you are doing it wrongly or it's not working. As much as I want to believe in magic, I know the imaginary magic wand doesn't just remove your burden from dieting and food rules. While diet instructions look like a coach yelling *shoulds* at you and blowing his whistle in your face, your Food Voice will always be flexible, kind, and nurturing.

A flexible Food Voice

When Rae considered how they would decide to eat, they first said, "When it is time"—following this up by saying that this included when they are hungry and are around friends gathered to eat a meal. Then Rae tried to take back that follow-up, noting they will only eat when hungry. The *shoulds* had countered Rae's initial Food Voice that eating should only happen when hungry.

Before we were taught to diet and distrust our food decisions, humans broke bread (or tortillas, rice, potatoes, naan, or many other cultural carbohydrate staples) to connect, feel pleasure, restore, and just eat! I believe Rae connected to this, yet their preprogrammed *I-Should-Eat* script got past security and busted into the guided imagery. It was triggered by flexibility.

The diet industry, with its foundation in racism, dictates perfectionistic, rigid rules. If you, like Rae, instinctually wrote you would eat when you're not hungry, you may have felt a painful response ping. This was actually a disconnect. It may have felt wrong or possibly even immoral. This is a part of your Food Voice needing attention.

Please gently inform that part of food's moral neutrality. Be compassionate with yourself because, like Rae, you were told food was either good or bad or healthy or unhealthy. Food has no morals to it because it is required to stay alive and is how we humans have always connected.

Food is flexible. Notice when your food thoughts gravitate toward black-and-white judgments. These classification systems came from the diet industry, not your Food Voice.

A kind Food Voice

We have become vigilant cautious eaters. We distrust ourselves around food especially if it tastes good, brings pleasure, and is satisfying. Some of the *shoulds* covering up your Food Voice are really wounded punishment scars. You may hear things like:

- "I can't buy chocolate because I will eat it when it's in my home."
- "I feel gross after eating that."
- "I only need one helping" (when you're eating your favorite meal served only on holidays).

Racism created authoritarian food rules out of thin air to control us. Do not minimize this intergenerational trauma: people have been killed for centuries to uphold racism's power. Your ancestors learned these food rules to survive and lovingly passed them on to you, hoping you will stay safe. Like a terrifying game of telephone, they learned over the centuries that staying slim symbolized a close relationship with the white, cisgender, thin ideal and gave access to power. The more power the safer one remains.

I have seen these oppressive systems translated into public health guidelines: the *USDA Dietary Guidelines for Americans, 2020–2025* states: "Enjoy a variety of foods, *but not too much*" (emphasis mine).[2] Over the last 30 years, public policy has focused on eating less, yet the USDA also informs us that one in five kids experiences hunger.[3] Forty-four million

Americans experience food insecurity, but US public policy continues to paint a picture of excess.

These oppressive systems have expected us to be okay with not getting the food we need. Pause when you hear distrust in your Food Voice. Consider instead that you are hearing one of your *I-Should-Eat* scripts programmed by one of these systems.

Your Food Voice will always kindly prioritize you getting enough food. It will always want to offer you one more in case you need it or want it. Your Food Voice will always encourage you to eat more food to help you recover from when you were told you couldn't or shouldn't.

Remember my client Paul whose dad's diabetes diagnosis changed his family's food choices and led to his feelings of food addiction? In a later session, I asked Paul to find a picture of his younger self before he struggled with a disallowing Food Voice. He brought a Polaroid straight from his family photo album. In it, younger Paul was hanging upside down at the playground, dangling by his legs waving his left hand at the camera. In his right hand he clutched a green football that he probably had been chasing around as evidenced by his flushed cheeks.

His mom told him he was about five in the picture and obsessed with throwing the football with his dad. Paul's dad had not yet been diagnosed with diabetes, and they still felt carefree with food.

Holding that picture, I took Paul through the Food Voice guided imagery again. I asked him to ask the same questions to five-year-old Paul and answer for him. His Food Voice immediately switched to a kind caretaker wanting him to have access to enough.

Sometimes, my clients didn't even feel a kind Food Voice looking at their younger self. Instead, they needed to picture their own child or a young child in their life. If you, too, struggle with hearing a kind Food Voice, consider visualizing a young person you care about. How would you want them to think about food? How much to eat? I hope this helps you peel back your scripts farther away from your Food Voice.

A nurturing Food Voice

Phrases like *food is medicine* strain my brain. While I appreciate eating certain nutrients can help us treat or prevent diseases, it doesn't have absolute power. Nutrition science trained us to believe absolutes like one bite of an egg causes heart disease until the message flipped to the heart-health-promoting effects of eating an egg every day. Add in oppressive systems and the amount of egg becomes a moot point anyway.

Yes, food does fuel us. It can be like a medicine, especially if we have not eaten enough. Calories give us energy to think, play, and move about. Calories wiggle our gastrointestinal tract to digest. Calories give us energy to move our diaphragm to help us breathe. Without eating enough, we do run out of fuel.

But food is so much more than the calories it provides. I remember eating a big bowl of leftover spaghetti and meatballs the morning after the 2016 US presidential election. Holding my warm navy Fiestaware bowl, I felt soothed by that eating experience. I felt hopeless, and swirling my fork through the saucy spaghetti disconnected me for a few moments from despair. The hot steam engulfing my face felt like the embrace I needed in that moment. I was eating emotionally, and that was a part of listening to my Food Voice.

Most intuitive eating coaches I see on social media discourage emotional eating. Along the way intuitive eating has been funneled into eating when hungry and stopping when full. This rigid rule blocks us from normal coping strategies.

If you and I were amoebas in an agar-filled Petri dish, eating only when hungry would probably be just fine. But we don't live in a Petri dish. We live outside those circular plastic walls and have seasons, time zones, different languages and customs, political parties with different beliefs, climate change, wars, weddings, divorces, new life, and death. Being a human is complicated as fuck. We are not robots, but live a complex human experience. Food as medicine only sets us up to fail because it ignores our complex humanity.

Your Food Voice includes a way to help you cope with life's different experiences. We eat at weddings and funerals for a reason, and it's not because we are addicted to food. Rather, food soothes and nurtures our emotions. Food moves serotonin with one bite. This is your strength, not your weakness.

Weave together different parts of your Food Voice

You've done so much work uncovering your Food Voice. Review how you answered the journal prompts throughout this chapter. Spend time holding all these new personal truths. I know you have a long complicated history with food and have felt the heavy burden from that relationship.

I find it helpful to try to gather all that you have now discovered and try to hold them figuratively at once. I often picture each individual nuance to your Food Voice as a strand of yarn. Framing food and body in this new way leads you to many new strands of *knowing* that don't feel familiar, even though they have always been there. These are the particulars of *your* Food Voice. I want you to notice the complexity and function of every single strand. I want you also to notice which oppressive systems impact your ability to connect with a kind, nurturing, and flexible Food Voice.

I hope you see now why I could not just type out these particulars for you. You had to discover them on your own because they are unique to you.

Build your Voice Finder Cord

I want this book to be more than just words going into your brain. I hope it changes your life! You have the power to get out of the Diet Trap using your Food Voice to permanently change how to connect to your scripts. Even more, with every step you make away from the Diet Trap, you help others get out, too.

To make this a reality, it's time to build your own Voice Finder Cord. This will be a visual reminder of your unique Food Voice and its past, present and future wishes. Just as one braids hair or a friendship bracelet, imagine weaving each aspect of your Food Voice strands so you can see it all together. Up and down, over and over, you notice food's satisfaction, fuel, pleasure, connection, intergenerational loops to ancestors passing along knowledge of recipes, missteps, soothing powers, and so much more.

With each passing strand, you notice how some spots are more wounded than others. Even though they may be painful, these wounded parts still provide you with innate wisdom—probably even more than those that have never bothered you before.

Go to FindYourFoodVoiceBook.com or library.johnmurraylearning. com to get more detailed instructions and a special bonus I've designed for you. I also have a coloring sheet to help you go through this exercise if the act of weaving is inaccessible or not desirable to you.

Step 1

Gather nine 24-inch-long pieces of yarn or string. Three strands need to be in the green color family, three in the blue color family, and three in the purple color family.

Step 2

Gather all nine pieces together and measure 2 inches down from the top. Tie a simple knot at around this 1-inch mark to gather them all together. This is your Voice Finder Knot symbolizing your unique relationship and history with food. Your magic wand guided imagery showed you a glimpse into your Food Voice, and this knot will help remind you of its constant presence. Even when you can't quite feel it, your Voice Finder Knot is always holding everything together.

Step 3

Separate the string into their three color families representing the three aspects of your Food Voice guiding you:

- **Blue:** Symbolizes the flexibility.
- **Green:** Symbolizes the kindness.
- **Purple:** Symbolizes the nurture.

Step 4

Gather the flexibility (blue) strands and braid them however you like. The braid can be as simple or as intricate as you see fit. As you are weaving the flexible parts of your Food Voice, say these statements out loud or in your thoughts:

- Food is morally neutral. It is neither good nor bad.
- My Food Voice does not have an absolute right or wrong next step in making my next food decision.
- When I struggle connecting with my Food Voice, I ask: "How can I be flexible?"

After you have woven your flexibility braid about 1 inch, tie a knot.

Next, gather the kindness (green) strands and braid them however you like. The braid can be as simple or as intricate as you see fit. As you are weaving the kind parts of your Food Voice, say these statements out loud or in your thoughts:

- My Food Voice prioritizes getting enough food.
- My Food Voice wants to offer one more in case I need it or want it.
- My Food Voice encourages me to eat more food to help me recover from when I was told I couldn't or shouldn't.
- When I struggle connecting with my Food Voice, I ask: "What is the kind choice?"

After you have woven your kindness braid about 1 inch, tie a knot.

Finally, gather the nurture (purple) strands and braid them however you like. The braid can be as simple or as intricate as you see fit. As you are weaving the nurture parts of your Food Voice, say these statements out loud or in your thoughts:

- My Food Voice helps me cope with life.
- My Food Voice wants food for energy, pleasure, connection, and emotional regulation. All these wants make me a successful human.
- When I struggle connecting with my Food Voice, I ask: "Am I nurturing my unmet needs?"

After you have woven your nurture braid about 1 inch, tie a knot.

Step 5

Repeat Step 4 and weave each strand however you like. As you are doing each one, consider these prompts for each section:

- **Blue: Your Past** This strand represents the food beliefs, customs, and experiences that your ancestors experienced. Some of these you may know and many you will not yet still live within you. Let your brain imagine their collective Food Voices and what they have wanted to pass down to you—whether those are helpful now or not.
- **Green: Your Present** What oppressive systems do you experience? Name them as you braid. Recognize their massive power. Notice how you have been manipulated to not see them. See which systems you contribute to upholding and can change for the better.

- **Purple: Your Future** What do you want to make different looking ahead? When you hold your magic wand and consider the possibilities, how do you want to relate to food? To your body? To movement? To others? As you braid, repeat these future wishes and imagine them already complete.

Step 6

After you have woven each individual Voice Finder Cord about another inch, tie a knot. This knot represents what is not yours: shame and blame. As you tie the knot, say this out loud: "*I-Should-Eat* scripts don't work for me because I am a successful human. This blame is no longer mine to carry."

When you hold all of your food history woven together, is it heavy or light? Simple or complex? Whatever you are holding right now, it is beautiful because it is all your own. Your Voice Finder Cord is a visual representation to remind you of your always present Food Voice even when outside forces build scripts to work against it.

Great work! You have started your Voice Finder Cord. We will continue to build this external version of your Food Voice throughout the rest of the book.

Moving on with Your Food Voice

Now that a part of you has experienced a few moments with your Food Voice and has a tangible representation of it, let's figure out how you want to integrate it with your reality. You have connected with something beautiful that cannot be taken away—your collected data containing feelings, thoughts, experiences, pictures, messages, or a combination of these. You have learned how to know when to eat, how to know when it feels best to stop depending on certain circumstances, what to include in your food choices, and what needs are met with eating. With time, I hope you come back to these vital Food Voice concepts—and remember yours is always kind, nurturing, and flexible. As you get to know it, you will add more details to it. I picture you like a sculptor, chipping away at the marble—not to create something but rather to reveal what has always been there.

While a part of you experienced your Food Voice, there lives a part of you that did not. Let's consider this as your *parallel self*. Your parallel self did not see the wand and its intricate carvings, didn't feel its weight or magic. It remains fully stuck in the diet industry and all of its systems of oppression.

What is the first thing you want this parallel part of you to know about your Food Voice?

What did you discover?

Spend time letting your parallel self know what he/she/they need to know. Go to FindYourFoodVoiceBook.com or library. johnmurraylearning.com to get a special worksheet I've designed to collect your thoughts.

Notice some parts of the braid need more attention compared to others. I find those spots uncover a painful history, and we will tend to them in later chapters. In the end, those spots will give you the greatest insight moving forward. They will keep you from getting sucked back into the Diet Trap.

Dear Kayla

Let's take a moment to pause and reflect. You've done so much work even though you don't feel productive. Want to know some secret insight? The diet industry keeps you focused on an outcome and "being productive." That's the trap. Can you slow things down and compassionately honor the pain among all the confusion? You are repairing your complicated history with food and not doing anything wrong. Diet culture and trauma have you thinking you're trapped because of your weakness. They are wrong! You've been in your strength all along. Your Food Voice wants to remind you that it is always kind, nurturing, and flexible. Honor that wisdom always there, and be compassionate with yourself when you disconnect from it.

Love,
Food

> ## Dear Food letter activity
>
> Write a letter to Food describing what it was like for you to connect with your Food Voice. Whether you connected for a moment or hours, describe what you know to be true so far about your innate ability to make food and movement choices.

References

1 Hirschmann, J. R. (2010). *When Women Stop Hating Their Bodies*. Ballantine Books.
2 https://www.dietaryguidelines.gov/sites/default/files/2020-12/DGA_2020-2025_ExecutiveSummary_English.pdf (accessed April 25, 2024).
3 https://www.ers.usda.gov/topics/food-nutrition-assistance/food-security-in-the-u-s/ (accessed April 25, 2024).

4

Tend

Dear Food,

When I was around 13 my mother told me that I needed to watch out because too much of you would take me to the "misses sizes"—which in that day was more like plus size. If I ate more of you than she felt happy with, she would give me a look of disappointment. I would sometimes whip up a bowl of cookie dough while she was out of the house, wolf you down, and then clean up as fast as possible.

Anyway, so from there I restricted and binged you. I went from diet fad to diet fad. Of course, I would get so many compliments from people when they observed my eating less of you, even when I was nearly starving myself. But those diets never lasted. I'd always come back to you, eat so much of you that you would make me sick. I'd swear never to binge on you again, but I always did.

My ups and downs with you have cost me so much money, Food! Between all the diets, special ingredients, and clothing… oh my… I cannot even imagine how much money I've wasted over these years trying to get to that size where I would be acceptable to my mother and, therefore, myself and others.

I was once again failing at keeping weight off during my most recent diet when I was introduced to intuitive eating, diet culture, and peace with food for the first time—wow—totally new concepts for me. I love them, and I want to incorporate them into my life. I so want peace with you and with myself! I want to accept where I am right now, at this moment!

However, I am discouraged and feeling confused. I have given myself freedom with all foods, and I've tried to eat only when I'm hungry and to stop when I'm full, but I have just gotten fatter, and that scares me. What is the normal process? Is this how it works? Is my body holding on to everything thinking I'll starve it again? Does it get worse before getting better? I want my journey towards loving you to be free and peaceful. Thanks for keeping me alive, Food. We just need to figure out how this relationship is going to pan out!

Love,
Time to DTR (define the relationship)

Let's unpack your suitcase

I greet you at my office door and show you into my therapy room. You sit on the green couch and that's when I notice your very heavy suitcase. You keep it hidden at first, yet when you sit down, the suitcase lands on the floor with a thud. I see you trying not to make a big deal about how heavy it is and hear you apologize for dropping it.

The suitcase barely stays shut, so jammed full is it with a mismatch of tough-to-contain memories, BMI printouts, WW point trackers, and empty diet drink cans. I see the shattered hope trying to hold it all together.

As we chat about the weather, you try to minimize how much space you and the suitcase take up. You apologize for its beat-up appearance and fib about where it has been. You make excuses for the suitcase like you caused all its clutter and deserve to have more burdens put inside it.

You want me to believe the suitcase has nothing to do with why we meet. Rather, you sing the suitcase's praises as if reading memorized lines from a script thrown at you so long ago. The suitcase is how you will find health someday, you say, and you hope I will add another token. I see another string of hope ready to tie things together.

I ask if you want to unpack what is in the suitcase. I want to help you sort through everything and make sense of it. I won't rush, I promise. I won't preach either.

You baulk at my attention to the suitcase's power over you. I am not supposed to see all of its contents together, rather just the top layer and your effort to keep meeting a goal. You show me how well you are following the directions. You wonder if I can just keep it light; you want me to not pry into the depth of the suitcase. Instead, you want me to stay on the surface and give you another directive script. It is easy for me to see all the scripts already there. How can I add anything different?

You decide it is okay to take out all the previously held scripts in your suitcase. Some are marked with points or macros or calories or exercise directions. Each journey began with hope for something better. At first, you connect with the longing for improved health and energy. Then, as we lay out all the open scripts, side by side, you notice something you have never seen before.

Each script disguised as a map says the final destination provides permanent acceptance, peace, and light. We study each one and name how they are all full of overpromises that underdeliver.

Each and every map had one final destination: isolating shame.

This realization brings tears to your eyes. Each script symbolizes your unmet needs and more pain. Each script brought more *shoulds*. Seeing them all laid out, you can't believe you've been carrying it all along by yourself for so long.

I wish you knew that suitcase full of diet history is not your individual burden. I see your shame trying to cover its tracks, yet still hoping it will provide.

How many more maps to the same destination do you need? I want you to know you have tried enough times. I *will* you to know this, too.

You have been tricked to believe you need an *I-Should-Eat* script. You don't. You just need your breath, noticing it rhythmically grounding you to meet your needs.

We fill the therapy room with all of your suitcase contents. You feel overwhelmed seeing it all now, wondering if it can still be packed up. It all feels too much.

We can go through this any way you want. We can leave it out and take our time looking at each piece with a magnifying glass. We can light a match and burn it all. We can group like with like, and name each era for what it means now.

Keep this in mind: you are in charge and there are no wrong ways moving forward. It is okay if it feels scary, sad, exhilarating, terrifying, or puzzling. It is okay to take breaks. You may feel alone, but you never are. It's not just me here. Look around at all of us sorting through our baggage not knowing how we got here and unsure about what is next.

Except now we are on our own terms.

Are you ready to move away from diets and the number on the scale as a measure of progress?

Finding your Food Voice means coming to terms with the fact that diets don't work and that your weight has zero to do with your worth. Only you know if you are truly ready to move away from the seductive *I-Should-Eat* scripts pulling you back to the Diet Trap. I don't think you've been given enough say in what you and your body have had to endure in your life so far. I want you to know you deserve body autonomy, even now when you're making the decision whether to diet or not.

Where are you on this decision? Ready? Or ambivalent? Or nowhere close?

This chapter is all about you and your personal history with food. This will help you clarify if you are ready and give you the rocket fuel to make the big steps out of your Diet Trap. A side note as we sift through your eating history: not every *I-Should-Eat* script comes from a diet. Let's include here any cue that manipulates food or your body in your eating history. Also, going through your food and body history can connect with difficult times in your life and even trauma, so give yourself space and compassion.

What emotions come up for you?

Consider for a moment that tomorrow will be the first day you will have when you don't rely on *I-Should-Eat* scripts. Which thoughts or feelings come to you first? Is there a pang of excitement? Freedom? Fear?

Sitting with those first thoughts and feelings, what comes to the surface next? Regret? Sadness? Hopelessness? Joy?

Matilda, my college age client with PCOS, described a quick rush of excitement picturing her future without dieting. As fast as that feeling came, it disappeared, as she imagined navigating her college campus— where there were very few plus-size students. If she stopped weighing herself, would she gain more weight? She looked down in a daze and told me how hard the school cafeteria would be as a higher-weight person not choosing a salad. Everyone was health obsessed and skinny at her school; not dieting would be radical. Sorting through all of this, Matilda said she was afraid to leave her Diet Trap.

Please do not ignore any emotions or thoughts while you and your brain get used to the idea of rejecting your scripts. Name these messages and ask them to join you in this process. I know these thoughts and emotions come from your lived experiences and inform your next steps.

Unpacking your *I-Should-Eat* scripts one at a time

Let's roll up our sleeves and get down to business. First order of business? Unpacking each and every *I-Should-Eat* script in your suitcase. Grab your worksheet for this section at FindYourFoodVoiceBook.com or library.johnmurraylearning.com.

Scripts come from:

- planned diets that restrict certain nutrition items like calories, carbs, fats, or food types
- healthy eating challenges that encourage you to limit certain foods and eat only from a preapproved list. This could be something that started out as "just eating organic" or "eating no processed food" or something like that
- family-of-origin food rules like "always clean your plate" or "the men in the family eat more"
- food rules that help you fit in at work, in your family, or within your community to help lessen racism, ableism, homophobia, anti-fat bias, transphobia, or other forms of oppression.

Each seductive *I-Should-Eat* script whispers in your ear. Because most people have learned dozens of scripts or more—that's a lot of confusing noise! We need to spend time focusing on each one; breaking each down will contribute to breaking its spell. This future reference provides a permanent remembrance of how futile each script was in your life. Take care of this process because you will reference these often while finding your Food Voice.

I appreciate how painstakingly slow this part of finding your Food Voice will be. Please don't skip these next steps. Spelling out the good, the bad, and the ugly of each script helps you get out of the Diet Trap.

How many *I-Should-Eat* scripts have you been on?

Do you know your number? Instinctively you probably have a number in mind that fits on one hand, yet I encourage you to think through this more. Rae had been on many diets since early childhood, so they knew their number was high, upwards of 30 or more. Paul, on the other hand, thought he really hadn't been on any diets because he never called them diets. As I described to him, just because an eating plan is not referred to as a diet doesn't mean it's not causing strain on your Food Voice.

To help Paul discern between his Food Voice and diets, we came up with a definition. Diets, we decided together, were a set of rules whose goal was to manipulate food choices to change the body's weight or health status. Remember, middle-school Paul's Food Voice got hit by his first *I-Should-Eat* script when his dad got diagnosed with diabetes. At that time, food was a way to manipulate his dad's blood sugar yet quickly evolved into a moral choice.

How would you define a diet in your life? There may be descriptions missing using Paul's definition. Note your nuanced definition in a journal, with permission to add to or subtract from this as you move along discovering your Food Voice.

How many scripts have you counted in your lifetime so far? Share your number on social media using #FoodVoice.

Your *I-Should-Eat* script timeline

Rae's first diet began with a pediatrician plotting their weight on the pediatric growth chart. That was easy for Rae to discern, yet from there things lost clarity. It was tough for Rae to know when their thoughts came from their own innate wisdom or when from a learned diet. Rae knew that deciphering each individual diet would help them untangle the *I-Should-Eat* script from their own Food Voice. While naming each diet will feel tedious, it will help you know which messages are your own and when they arise from diet industry manipulation.

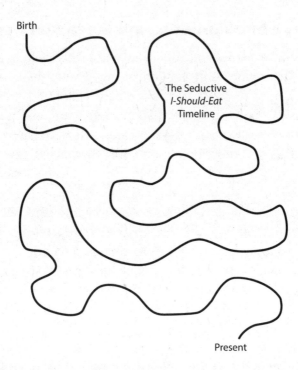

Birth

The Seductive
I-Should-Eat
Timeline

Present

Using a graphic like this one, Rae and I spent a session mapping out each diet, which often coincided with significant life experiences like starting puberty, coming out, first partner, summer camp, leaving for college, breakups, miscarriage, divorce, and death. We also were sure to include any oppressive systems Rae experienced. For example, Rae noticed many drastic diets took place while gaining clarity on their trans masculine gender identity; seeing this, they could name how transphobia gave diets tremendous power.

After putting this diet history timeline together, Rae left the session believing they included every *I-Should-Eat* script. Then they went home and looked at some old scrapbooks from childhood and early adulthood. Seeing the visual representation of their memories brought even more scripts to the fore, and we added them to Rae's timeline. See Rae's completed timeline as well as ones from other Voice Finders mentioned at FindYourFoodVoiceBook.com or library.johnmurraylearning.com. I hope these examples help you as you move to the next step in finding your Food Voice: building your *I-Should-Eat* scripts timeline.

As you build your timeline, be kind to yourself, as you may need many attempts to remember every single detail. Part of each script's job is to try to shield you from pain especially when it comes to oppressive systems. You may not remember every single script today. It's okay if you go back to add more scripts as you move forward with this book.

Something else to keep in mind, while building this timeline: I expect emotions to come up including sadness, shame, guilt, anger, or despair. Tapping into your history will brush against old wounds that haven't healed. Take your time and take breaks when you need them. Remind yourself often you are not broken, but functioning within oppressive systems. Rediscovering how to eat without these scripts will keep you out of your Diet Trap, promote health, and help set others free.

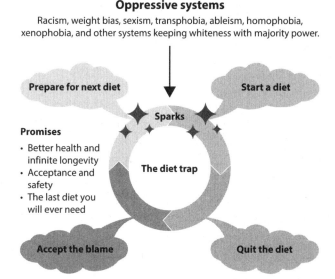

Oppressive systems
Racism, weight bias, sexism, transphobia, ableism, homophobia, xenophobia, and other systems keeping whiteness with majority power.

Prepare for next diet

Start a diet

Sparks

Promises
- Better health and infinite longevity
- Acceptance and safety
- The last diet you will ever need

The diet trap

Accept the blame

Quit the diet

Catalog each *I-Should-Eat* script

Now that you have a list of all the scripts on your timeline with room to add more as they pop into your consciousness, we need to break each one down. Doing this will help you pivot away from all of them in the next chapter. It will be hard work and good work.

We need to gather more details to help you gain clarity on why each script harmed you, how they helped you, and how to avoid them in the future. This is another part of the finding your Food Voice process where I am afraid I may lose you. This is a tedious step, yet it will help you uncover what you need to get out of the Diet Trap forever. Take breaks if you need it—yet stay with me!

Go to FindYourFoodVoiceBook.com or library.johnmurraylearning.com to get your worksheet; each script will get its own page.

Name the spark

All scripts start with a spark of hope. Remember, these sparks are all reel-you-back-in seductive fantasies. This hope perpetuates each script's manipulation, keeping you stuck in the Diet Trap.

First, let's answer: What was the promise with each script you started? Maybe it promised to be your last diet and a permanent solution for your weight or health. Other fantasies promised a health cure for diabetes or PCOS. See Rae's answer below. They started a low-carb diet the summer after graduating from high school. Looking toward their next phase of life, they wanted to look their best starting college. Rae recalled the fear of rejection and wanting so much to find a group of friends and fit in. The low-carb diet promised Rae acceptance, ease, and more friends.

List the short-term outcomes

Weight and nutrition research suggests all diets improve health and promote weight loss in the short term. How did this script, too? Was it predictably delivering on its promise in the short term? The Diet Trap keeps you stuck because of how successful diets are in this short term—this gives scripts all the credit yet none of the blame.

Ignoring these short-term outcomes just keeps a script stronger. Let's not contribute to its strength, rather let your lived experiences dissolve its power.

Rae recalled the low-carb diet helped them go down two clothing sizes which excited Rae and their mom. Rae remembered their mom was so happy buying them new clothes as a reward. Rae smiled big and bright just recalling the shopping trip. It was apparent to me that the weight loss brought Rae and mom closer, something that Rae needed during that time of life.

Which system of oppression contributed to this *I-Should-Eat* script?

Scripts are seductive because oppressive systems control their puppet strings. Consider the oppressive systems discussed in Chapter 2 and others you know about. Which of these systems did this particular script go to bat for?

Rae easily identified anti-fat bias as a reason they started the low-carb diet before leaving for college. Rae recalled a constant fear of rejection from peers, family, and strangers because of their body size. Doing this diet helped them feel hopeful they would find acceptance.

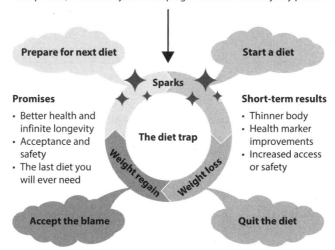

Oppressive systems

Racism, weight bias, sexism, transphobia, ableism, homophobia, xenophobia, and other systems keeping whiteness with majority power.

Rae knew they were not cisgender in high school, yet did not feel safe vocalizing that until much later when they were in college. Looking back, Rae noted how homophobia and transphobia were systems working against their Food Voice and strengthened their resolve to follow the low-carb diet plan.

Finding your Food Voice is tough because of these systems. Just like everything else in this process, ignoring their role will only strengthen their grip on you. Because I don't hold the same identities as many of the people I have worked with, I cannot understand what it is like to live with these systems and work against them. This goes for you as well. I do know, though, you can connect to your Food Voice. This connection starts by you naming the harmful systems impacting you and removing yourself as the blame.

What did the script actually bring long-term?

Diets have gotten enough kudos; it's time to get back to long-term reality.

Rae's smile quickly faded as they recalled struggling with food that first semester in college. Rae said they declined invitations to meet up with new dorm friends because they involved pizza. They didn't trust themselves to say no to pizza, so Rae ate a low-carb meal replacement bar in their room alone.

Most of the time, Rae explained, this led to binge eating in the cafeteria. What did this low-carb diet really bring Rae?

- missing out on friendships
- shame
- isolation
- obsessing over food choices
- binge eating
- weight cycling (Rae's weight by the end of the first semester was two dress sizes higher than before starting the diet).

Generally, possible long-term outcomes include:

- restriction, bingeing, purging, or other eating disorder behaviors
- worsened health
- depression
- anxiety
- social isolation
- food obsession
- weight cycling (weight loss then regain then gain even more than lost)
- strained relationships
- more chaotic and complicated relationship with food
- more time thinking about food and body
- blame and shame for the diet not working.

This list is not exhaustive—I know I have missed many long-term outcomes. Rae found themselves going through college scrapbooks and journals to help them recall each long-term script consequence.

Rae admitted it took too much from their college experience and kept them from really getting to know the adult they were becoming. Rae angrily cried recalling all of this. We heard my front-office door chime open as Rae was drying their tears. We both took a deep breath knowing there was so much work to be done because college was 20 years ago for Rae!

"This is such hard work," Rae said. "I know I have barely scratched the surface but cataloging each script, I feel more affirmed in my decision to stop dieting."

"Exactly," I said. "This is hard, and going through each one will be ammo to fuel your pivot away from their seductive fantasy. You are doing a great job at this. Do you want to meet next week or take a break?"

Rae countered, "Oh no, diets will not take more time. What do you have open next week?"

Over the next few weeks, Rae and I filled out *I-Should-Eat* script worksheets on each diet they could recall. I encourage you to do the same. Just like Rae, it will be the ammo to help you pivot. The diet industry's invisible veil over society takes tremendous energy to reject. You need all the ammo you can get as we get you set to pivot. Onward!

Dear Time to DTR,

We see you trying to make peace yet at the same time struggle with acceptance. Your relationship with Food was founded on the white, cis, thin ideal. As you mend your body image, consider collecting all of your lived experiences with diets. Each diet created a *I-Should-Eat* script whispering in your ear. How did they start? What were their promises? Did they deliver? What did they ultimately bring? We know you are struggling with relying on your body and know you may find a different way that fits for you. Your history will inform your next steps toward peace. We are so proud of the healing work you are doing. We are with you on this journey.

Love,
Food

Dear Food letter activity

Write a letter to Food naming all the short-term benefits you got from your *I-Should-Eat* scripts. Describe how these deceived you into believing the script was the solution and kept you as the blame when the long-term consequences emerged. Call out these negative outcomes and remind yourself you never needed to be fixed.

Voice Finder Cord activity

Hold the blue family of strings. Braid about an inch and consider your own personal suitcase like we heard about in the beginning of this chapter. How many *I-Should-Eat* scripts does it hold? After weaving about an inch, tie a knot and think about the estimated number of scripts you have tried. Gently rub this knot to remind yourself this is your data and insight that scripts will not work for you. This does not make you a failure; it makes you a successfully evolved human.

After braiding about an inch or two more, secure with a knot.

5

Pivot

Dear Food,

I know exactly when our journey began. I had an abnormally skinny ballerina body and had gained a few pounds over the summer. I knew what I had to do. My parents always did diets so I figured it was just a part of growing up.

Little did I know that losing those few pounds would lead to a horrible relationship with you and an unhealthy amount of weight gain. I used to not think about you. When I was bored, you weren't the first one I went to. You were fuel not an addiction. Never in a million years would I have thought I would be where I am now.

I have drifted so far and our relationship is so weak. I hate you but love you at the same time. You control me and I cannot contain myself around you. I'm addicted. You control my thoughts and take up my whole life. The more I pull away, the more I am attracted to you. I'm not sure why I go to you. Maybe it's my low self-esteem, or my body image issues, or my constant want and need to look like society's beauty standards. I feel that you are an escape; I have to run from my toxic thoughts about my body because no one else cares. I feel like I cannot even continue my daily life because of the hold you have on me. I hate myself because of you but I can't stop going back to you. I've tried to limit you but our relationship seems to get worse and worse. You were enjoyable, now I dread you. I'm fearful of what you will do to me. I'm fearful of how far I will go with you. You used to be a natural instinct that didn't matter to me, now I can't go five minutes without wanting you or thinking about how you ruin me.

I guess the truth is … you aren't the problem. It's me. I abuse you. I hate myself so I become overwhelmed and run to you. I'm not sure why I go to you. It seems counterproductive, but I'm in hopes of finding out why you have such a hold on me. I am guilty after going to you. I am humiliated, even if no one else knows. All I want is a healthy relationship with you and my body so I can move on with my life.

Sincerely, a girl who needs help

As we begin your pivot, I want to honor you and your commitment to repairing your Food Voice. I appreciate this has been hard work and you may have uncovered painful parts of your life. What's next? Expect concrete steps in this pivot to help you begin your Food Voice rebuild. Now it is on your terms.

Preparing to pivot

Relying on yourself to manage eating is scary especially if you've been following some sort of *I-Should-Eat* script for as long as you can remember. You may picture all-or-nothing scenarios—following a specific meal plan versus eating whatever whenever. Eating nothing versus eating everything. Being good versus being bad. Eating healthily versus unhealthily. My eyes feel the whiplash just thinking about the metaphorical tennis match between dieting and not dieting. It's the diet industry that has caused this dramatic black-and-white response to not following a script.

You have unconditional permission to eat whatever and whenever you want, *and* if this terrifies you, this chapter is written for you.

It does not have to be extreme. We can take our time.

Your scripts convinced you of these lies:

- Not dieting is losing control.
- You cannot trust yourself around food.
- Physical hunger cannot be trusted.
- Emotional eating is wrong.
- Your life goal is to stay a certain size, otherwise you are unlovable.

You've been walking a tightrope while being told you can't trust your own balance. You were made to hold on to heavy burdens that didn't even belong to you. Even though you have now set them aside, I see you are still on the tightrope and unfortunately just looked down for the first time.

You may picture other anti-diet folks doing a diet to food freedom 180-degree turnaround. It as though they have just jumped off the tightrope and are flying away without a care in the world. Wouldn't that be wonderful?

After 20 years I can let you know no one moves away from their complicated food history this way. Instead, people slowly and cautiously move away from their scripts. I often picture my clients tiptoeing away from a scary sleeping giant. Step by step, they try not to wake up the fiercesome troll. People rejecting their scripts for the first time tend to turn their head a few degrees to one side as they consider new options. They aim for them and make the first few shaky steps. As new options become truths, their stride quickens. A few even clang metal cooking pans, hoping to wake up the giant and gave it the middle finger.

You probably are not ready for making a loud exit from your *I-Should-Eat* scripts. This isn't a weakness. This is a strength. You have a lot to be skeptical about, after all!

While you are beginning to pivot, I just ask you to gently turn your head away from your complicated eating history and consider one tiptoe at a time away from your scripts. Remember that each movement forward, no matter how small, will help keep you out of the Diet Trap, promote health, and help set others free.

What are your *I-Should-Eat* script themes?

In Chapter 4, you tended to your complicated food history. You made a timeline and sifted through each script. This data steers you in the direction toward your Food Voice. Your collected information will be the compass to help you tiptoe away from relying on future scripts.

I encourage you to look at each cataloged script entry. As a visual person, I like to line up each page on a big table to get a bird's-eye view. Take a step back and consider them as a whole. Heads up: this can be a tough exercise, especially for the more recent scripts. Even tougher if you have experienced complex trauma. Working with a dietitian or another clinician, if accessible to you, can help you connect the dots.

Consider any repeating patterns. Noticing patterns will help you to know where to incorporate more guardrails and boundaries to protect your Food Voice. Themes often show up in these areas:

- reasons for starting a new script such as a health scare, milestone, or big event. You may notice similar sparks of hope for each script
- microaggression (or macroaggression) triggers from racism, anti-fat bias, ableism, etc.
- positive short-term diet wins like meeting a new romantic partner, getting a promotion, or being seen
- upticks in a mood disorder squashed in the short term by the script.

Certainly, Rae recognized that their desire to fit in and be liked was a big draw for them to start dieting. Remember their pediatrician even said dieting would enable them to have more friends. Rae felt so hopeful with each new script. *Be wary of these hopeful sparks*. Sparks feel *good* and they are so darn seductive. I encourage you to practice calling them out when they happen from now on. These moments of wonder and aspiration have tremendous power to block your Food Voice and healing journey. Name them in the moment for what they are—empty promises that don't work co-created by white supremacy and its diet industry minions.

There is an exception to this, of course. Rae was often misgendered before they started this journey to find their Food Voice. This transphobia along with constant anti-fat bias made starting a new diet a way to manage these oppressive systems. Rae said they fit into chairs with more ease and got less flack at the doctor's office after losing a certain amount of weight. Rae was safer when dieting especially in the short term.

I wish rejecting scripts was the same experience for every human. If you are cisgender and white and can buy clothes in just about any department store, your script sparks are blanket empty promises. They are lies. Your journey is not easy, for sure, and it's different. If you have an identity historically marginalized, well, things become more complicated. Rejecting your scripts will be radical and a heavier lift. Rejecting the diet industry can bring on more discrimination. I want you to know that those of us not experiencing as much oppression are working *with* you to change systems of oppression. This is not your individual burden. The only way for all of us to connect with our Food Voice is to help everyone connect with theirs.

What about health in the pivot?

As Matilda started her work to find her Food Voice, she worried about her health since she had PCOS. Would she be letting herself go? She was told to restrict carbs and sugar to lower her A1c (a blood test to give a graduated average of her blood sugar). She wondered whether, if she ate without a dos-and-don'ts list, she would ruin her health. Do you worry about this, too? Do you have a complicated history with food and a chronic condition managed by your eating?

Finding your Food Voice is complicated for everyone, and especially so if you have a chronic illness. This is key: prioritizing healing always promotes health.

Gentle nutrition and food hierarchy

Ellyn Satter, dietitian and therapist, writes about incorporating foods for health promotion as the last step in a hierarchy of needs for a healthy food relationship. What comes first? Consistently eating enough. Other steps include:

- access to enough acceptable food
- reliable ongoing access to food
- consistently satisfying food
- novel food experiences
- and last: instrumental food or food that modifies health.

Puzzled? Our healthcare visits frequently monitor eating choices rather than food access. I remember working in a hospital and being given doctor's orders to teach a patient heart-healthy eating. Upon reading this patient's medical record, I learned they lived with food insecurity because of unemployment. Teaching someone without enough food access how to eat less of certain foods and more of others is not only pointless, but also insulting. It misses the real issue: the patient's heart health and quality of life will be positively impacted by giving consistent access to food, any food, first.

This particular discharge diet instruction reminds me the diet industry does not treat us like humans but rather as useful workers upholding oppressive systems.

If you don't experience poverty, you may wonder if you can skip ahead to eating for health promotion. Consider other reasons for food insecurity: your *I-Should-Eat* scripts.

Matilda, while financially secure with open access to enough food at her university, did not have enough food. The anti-fat bias on campus prevented her from eating enough at meals. She felt uncomfortable eating a snack in front of others. When she told me how much she was eating and after reviewing her thorough food journals I knew she was not eating enough food.

I told Matilda that this may sound bizarre yet it is key: eating enough is *always* best. Our body does not like starvation and will do everything in its power to overcome consequences from it. It will slow down metabolism as well as mobilize (and increase) insulin, blood sugar, and cholesterol. In the short term, modifying food choices while not eating enough may improve some health markers. But Matilda, like you, was in it for the long game. Long term, not eating enough harms health. I told Matilda then, and I plead to you now, repairing your relationship with food to gain access to enough food will lead to long-term health improvements.

In a later chapter I will share with you ways to include foods to promote health improvements. Don't skip ahead. Those tools only help you find your Food Voice when other steps happen first.

Mental health versus physical health

When Paul described his eating potato chips in secret I immediately grew concerned about his emotional wellbeing. Not surprisingly, he shared that he had feelings of shame, despair, and hopelessness whenever his brain felt obsessed with food. He said he felt isolated and depressed.

> Mental health is physical health. Research finds connection with mental health and higher blood sugar, cardiovascular disease, and other chronic health conditions.[1]

When you prioritize healing your history with food, you *are* prioritizing your health. You are not giving up, rather actively working toward improving health. Witnessing this work, I know it is neither easy nor passive. Remember, it is hard work and good work.

Future *I-Should-Eat* script temptations

As you begin the pivot away from your *I Should Eat* scripts, the temptation to go back to them will be high. It is important to honor any positives that have come from diets, rigid eating behaviors, or any food rules. Because you have tried so many scripts, you can probably predict now what the short-term outcomes will be if you tried again. You don't need to try another script to see if those short-term outcomes are different; you have tried enough.

Consider all your gathered script inventory from that bird's-eye view again. Do you notice a collective long-term result from them? What were your common patterns? If you tried a new script, would the long-term outcome change? I hope you have clarity that the answer is no. Have you tried enough to predict long-term outcomes? I think you have.

Rejecting the diet industry challenges us because of the complexity of positive short-term outcomes versus the dangerous yet not apparent until much later long-term outcomes. I encourage you to remind yourself of this when you feel that spark of hope from both the short- *and* long-term outcomes.

I want you to document these newly found script patterns and themes. Go to FindYourFoodVoiceBook.com or library.johnmurraylearning.com to get a worksheet I created for you or jot down the following in a notebook:

- the sparks that get you started
- the short-term results that keep you fooled
- the inevitable long-term results that you blame on yourself.

This is *the* document to keep handy. Stick it on your mirror and read when brushing your teeth. Make a screenshot to use as your phone's wallpaper. Keep it within arm's reach while you are finding your Food Voice. When you are tempted to start a new diet or try a different way to manipulate your body weight, reference your Patterns and Themes document. It is your proof from your own data that those scripts—no matter how flashy new ones will be—don't work for you.

Your pivot begins with guardrails

Have you tried to move away from your scripts before? For many, the experience is incredibly chaotic. I have lost count of the people who read *Intuitive Eating* on their own and, while excited, freaked out after a few weeks. When you have been relying on a list or set of orders to make eating decisions, your body and mind flail. Those first few moments away from your scripts can be terrifying and exhausting.

Whenever Paul took away a food rule, he felt addicted to food. He said food felt like an obsession when not dieting. He described constant food noise in his head. Food rules gave him a calm feeling and the bandwidth to do his job. He could take care of himself. The mere thought of bringing pastries, cookies, and chips home brought fearful tears to his eyes. "How can I learn how to trust my Food Voice when I am terrified? It feels impossible to just eat whatever I want when I want. I know I will binge."

Bingeing or out-of-control eating experiences occur as you are finding your Food Voice. Have you experienced more of them while reading this book? It is okay and I will discuss ways through this in a later chapter. For now, keep in mind binges or other out-of-control eating experiences don't mean you are doing anything wrong. An uptick in binges signals repair is happening.

However, I appreciate this is a great example of "easier said than done."

If you have never-ending bandwidth or time, you can remove any *I-Should-Eat* script and let your mind and body heal in these binges. Like a pendulum pulled farther back, it will swing to the opposite side with as much gusto. Eventually, though, with time moving back and forth, the pendulum will swing with less energy behind it. The human experience of not eating enough (from any script) pulls that pendulum back. Letting go and letting it swing often provokes a binge. As it swings back and forth, over time it eventually has a calmer less energetic pull in both directions.

No time for violent pendulum swings? Paul didn't either.

Paul wondered if the GLP-1 weight-loss medications, like Ozempic or Wegovy, were his answer to out-of-control eating experiences. He had read how people noticed their food noise disappearing as they ramped their dosage up. Paul asked his doctor if he would be a candidate for it and she quickly handed him a prescription. She thought he could lose some weight. Before filling out the prescription—something he would have to pay out of his own pocket for—his partner Gene encouraged him to meet with me to discuss.

While I have my own opinions on GLP-1s for weight loss and food noise, this was not my decision. We made pro and con charts, and ultimately Paul decided to wait on starting the injections. He decided to first give a different plan a try, yet reserved the right to change his mind.

Paul didn't want to experience these exhausting binges anymore. If you, too, are not up for violent pendulum swings, we have a plan.

I told Paul we can continue working through his complicated history with food using a concept I call *guardrails*. I picture these guardrails as a set of props you might see in a yoga class. Instead of going straight into the full yoga pose expression, props like blocks and straps help people access each pose. Laura Burns, author of *Big and Bold: Yoga for the Plus Size Woman*, uses yoga props from the start. She says this invites more people to access each pose and build from there.

Guardrails are like yoga props. I, like Laura, start with guardrails when I introduce non-diet ways of eating. Why not give more people a chance to find their Food Voice? Going straight into intuitive eating or any other non-diet technique will be accessible only for a few people.

You have a number of guardrails to pick from and some may be better suited for you than others. You may need just one or may need them all. I encourage you to refrain from judging yourself for using these guardrails. There is nothing wrong with using them, and I find they help the mind experience less chaotic feelings or noise around food and body. Scripts promote food preoccupation and these guardrails help your body practice having more space in your thoughts *not* given over to food.

Guardrails also help the body repair from the years of scripts. You have been programmed to not trust yourself around food; guardrails help you get reacquainted with your innate kind, flexible, and nurturing Food Voice.

Start with check-in props (CHIPS)

Paul described himself as a food addict, and I considered him to be preoccupied with food. In Chapter 2 I described why humans become food preoccupied as an evolved trait to keep us alive. You may have tried on your own to move away from your scripts but found your brain overwhelmed with loud food thoughts. This is exhausting and keeps you stuck in the Diet Trap.

When your brain is used to thinking about food all the time, it will keep thinking about food all the time until your body's internal systems trust you will continue to have access to enough food. You also need practice having gentle space in your brain to not think about food. While there is no way to predict how long this will take, I have found *check-in props*, or CHIPS for short, help the brain practice relaxing its thoughts about food in short bursts.

I first learned this check-in procedure via Christopher Fairburn's cognitive behavioral research. Some of his methodology has a weight focus so I have adapted it to be weight inclusive. What I learned from his research was that the food-preoccupied brain, over time, becomes used to food thoughts. These thoughts have strong neural pathways and default to always thinking about food. Food obsession becomes the brain's preferred way to function.[2]

Think of your brain's food thoughts to be like a well-paved Los Angeles superhighway. Always crowded with cars zooming. If you try to take an exit but traffic is too fast and tight, you can easily miss it.

The CHIP pause

To help your brain learn how to have space again without food preoccupation you need two things: enough food throughout the day and practice check-ins to reassure your brain that you are ready to give it enough food. These function as a literal yield sign for that superhighway.

This pause helps you look around and decide what to do next. At each CHIP, I encourage you to go through a series of steps to ground yourself, then ask yourself a series of questions.

Step 1: Ground

At each CHIP, pause electronics, put down your pen, and place your feet on the ground. If you can, open a window or get yourself outside. I find that, if you can connect with outside air, this helps even more.

Begin by connecting with your breath. Feel it go in and notice your chest rise. Hold it for a moment and try to count to four. Let your air release and notice your chest lower. Hold for four more seconds.

Go through this breathing exercise four times. Some people like to also place their hands to feel their heartbeat like we did in the Food

Voice magic wand exercise. Picture that magic wand if you need to. Practice noticing your body working for you every single moment of every single day.

Step 2: Set the stage

Grab your Voice Finder Cord and notice the three necessary components to your Food Voice: kind, nurturing, and flexible. Your Food Voice is compassionate and curious. Your scripts are rigid and treat you like an asshole. Remind yourself these pause moments are meant to be free of judgment and notice when your thoughts align with your Food Voice and when they do not. At the end of this chapter, you will find directions on how to add CHIPs to your Voice Finder Cord.

Step 3: Ask barometer questions

CHIPs give you practice noticing how your mind and body are doing. The mind–body reconnection will help awaken and amplify your Food Voice. Your pause and stage setting move out clutter and dust to make way for your body and mind to rewire as a team. This rewiring and repair work happens each time you act as a barometer.

Barometers are scientific instruments used to predict weather. Metaphorically, they symbolize changes in your environment. While finding your Food Voice, these barometer questions will help you get to the information on whether or not changes have occurred within. Over time and with practice, you will begin to notice subtle cues requesting you to pay attention.

After grounding and setting the stage at your CHIP, ask these questions:

- Am I hot or cold?
- What am I feeling? Or, if this fits better, what messages am I getting from my brain?
- Do I need to use the bathroom?
- What are my thoughts focused on?
- Am I physically hungry? How do I know?
- Am I emotionally hungry? What does it symbolize?

Let's break down why each of these questions is important to run through within each CHIP.

CHIP barometer questions

Am I hot or cold?

Your Food Voice is kind and curious. Zooming into food questions can often get us back on that superhighway to food and body judgment. Starting with your temperature can be a safer segway into interoceptive awareness. Interoceptive awareness is the "ability to be aware of internal sensations in the body, including heart rate, respiration, hunger, fullness, temperature, and pain, as well as emotion sensations."[3] Unlocking this type of connection with your body, if you have access to it, can expedite Food Voice communication.

As you go through these questions, you may find interoceptive awareness inaccessible. Neurodivergent clients or those recovering from persistent trauma often experience different nuances to body connection. If this is you, you may have found hunger fullness scales and other intuitive eating tools unhelpful. You *can* find your Food Voice, but how you connect with it may just look different. That is okay! I encourage you to still ask these questions and answer them for *you*.

What am I feeling? Or, what messages am I getting from my brain?

Your barometer CHIPs help you to understand your thoughts and feelings. These thoughts and feelings are constantly churning and shifting yet, especially during busy times of your day, go unnoticed. I want you to practice checking in with them. This will help your mind–body connection rise to the surface and paint a picture of your present state of mind. Notice what feelings come up and practice being nonjudgmental about them. Not noticing a feeling? Shift the question to "What messages am I getting?"—this question can be especially helpful if you have trouble naming your feelings. After a few weeks checking in on this, you will notice a pattern to how your body communicates these shifts. This is gold. It can't be found in a diet book or good/bad food list. It is only within you.

Do I need to use the bathroom?

Check-in times aren't just about feelings. They are also practical, sometimes boring self-care. Just like hot versus cold, considering your unmet need to use the bathroom will be less judgmental. After all that work with feelings, shifting to another bodily function that doesn't get judged for its changing requests gives you insight to apply to your relationship with food. Do you ever restrict yourself to urinating only three times per day? If you need to pee more often, are you bad? Of course not. Your relationship with toilet work can be an example for how you will take care of eating: do it when your body tells you to, and don't think about it again until necessary.

What are my thoughts focused on?

You'll find your Food Voice when you can be in the here and now. Because you have these CHIPs throughout the day you will be doing different activities. Some of those activities may have food connections and some will not. Getting used to barometer checks during *all* activities will help your Food Voice come through in a variety of settings. This is important in your repair process. Have you noticed food thoughts swirling when relaxing in front of the TV but being disconnected from food thoughts while doing a work activity? Paul thought this meant he was only addicted to food while at home and "being good" was easier at work. I gently reminded Paul that distractions can be a part of self-care yet also a tool for the scripts. Practice acknowledging boring moments and charged moments during your CHIPs. This helped Paul get used to less of an all-or-nothing food pattern. Asking during his work day and when at home helped his mind–body wiring to get used to thinking about food *and* not thinking about food.

Am I physically hungry? How do I know?

When your food thought superhighway fires up at certain times of day or during particular activities, hunger may be easy to spot. But what about the rest of the day? Asking yourself many times throughout the day if you are hungry helps you look for your hunger signs. This part of CHIPs gets the most positive votes from previous clients, helping them to quiet the distractions and connect with physical hunger.

What is physical hunger? If you have this question, don't worry. You are not alone. The answer will vary. Checking in with these props will help you understand your hunger's language.

Kinds of hunger

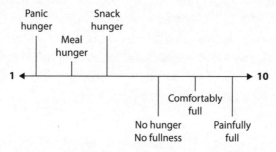

Hunger and fullness vocabulary

Hunger has different degrees of intensity. You may notice meal hunger is much more intense than snack hunger. As you are doing this activity in real time, note how it's different for you. Paul noticed his meal hunger interrupted his thoughts and made noises in his stomach. Snack hunger, on the other hand, felt more fleeting and gentler. He described it to be more like a tap on the shoulder rather than intense pangs in his stomach.

Reading through Paul's CHIP food journals, I saw a starred entry. When I asked him about it, Paul exhaled loudly and told me *that* meal hunger was different. It felt panicky and rushed. Reading through more of the entry I noted his penciled-in Binge ☹.

I looked at him and could feel his shame from across the room.

"You didn't do anything wrong, Paul," I said gently.

"But it felt wrong. I felt so calm and in control of my eating while doing those CHIPs. I was thinking I was cured but then I had a rushed lunch and a stressful afternoon in client mediation. By the time I got home I had my head in every pantry cabinet and just ate right out of the fridge. When I finally stopped eating I felt guilt and I also felt physically awful. In that moment I wanted to give up. But then I heard your voice telling me I can't do this wrong. To just notice. It all feels so easy until it isn't. What should I have done instead?"

I explained to Paul how important these experiences are to find your Food Voice. We need these experiences that feel like missteps—but aren't—to know how to take care of ourselves. "This is your data that informs you. I encourage you to notice the swirling judgment about what transpired yet try to not stay there. I wish these tough experiences didn't have to happen, but everyone needs them in order to figure out what they need." I asked him if it was okay to ask some follow-up questions and he nodded in approval.

"You mentioned you had a rushed lunch. Do you remember what you had?"

Paul told me it was a boxed catered lunch that had a chicken salad, apple, and a roll. "Thinking back, I remember working on that afternoon's mediation. I knew it would be stressful and didn't feel hungry at all. I tried to eat anyway because I knew I wouldn't be able to eat during the meeting. I think I picked at the salad and apple; I didn't eat the roll."

"Maybe that just wasn't enough food to get you through that meeting? Especially this stressful meeting?" I wondered out loud.

"But why did I lose my mind when I got home? I felt such an urgency to eat anything and everything. I remember thinking that I didn't have time to cook. I needed to just eat NOW. I truly felt an animal ripping open the cabinet doors," he said, shame coloring every word. "I felt so out of control."

It was so hard for him to admit this to me. These moments are close to the soul; it was protected information. "Paul," I said, "would you be okay if I shared some thoughts on this you may find helpful?"

"That is why I am here—help me stop doing this! I want to stop bingeing!" he pleaded.

"It sounds like in this moment your body and brain were overwhelmed with *panic hunger*. Panic hunger may feel out of control. Many call it binge eating. While I am not one to correct someone's description of their eating experiences, I think it's futile to pathologize something so normal and important for survival.

"You weren't doing anything wrong; rather you were being a successful human. When our bodies need food urgently, preparing a 'sensible meal'"—cue my eye roll—"won't cut it. You didn't lose your mind or control; rather your body was maintaining it. It sent you clear messages that eating was the absolute priority. Now I appreciate you did not like this experience and felt sluggish afterward. We can chat about options for next time this happens if you like."

Paul countered, "I don't want this to happen again. It took me days to recover mentally. I felt physically ill when I woke up the next morning like I was hung over."

I shared with Paul the seven important considerations in understanding panic hunger while finding your Food Voice:

1 Panic hunger is normal *when* your body doesn't get enough food and/or rest. Sometimes you can predict this and sometimes you cannot. When you notice panic hunger hitting, practice saying it out loud: *This is panic hunger.* Reassure yourself this is normal and you will be okay.

2 When you experience panic hunger, let yourself eat. Permission is key to healing. I encourage you to have plenty of ready-to-eat shelf-stable food that you enjoy and feels energizing to you especially during this CHIPs phase.

3 Resist the urge to allow only certain foods during panic hunger. Foods with positive diet culture messaging will leave you unsatisfied, stuck longer, and exhausted. Remember, prioritizing healing is healthy. Sometimes eating a cookie or chips or whatever is satisfying in that moment is the healthiest choice. I don't say this lightly: this is very important, while also easier said than done. It is normal for this to take lots of practice.

4 Reassure yourself after you stop eating that your response to panic hunger is an evolved human trait. This is absolutely not a weakness. You are being a successful human.

5 Once you feel calmer physically and emotionally, go through the last eight to twelve hours. Be curious and compassionate about your self-care: Did you have a stressful day? Did you give yourself enough food throughout the day? Did you take any breaks? This may be obvious like it was for Paul or it might not. Some of my clients need a number of panic hunger experiences to find themes.

6 Use this new data moving forward. Experiment with implementing more self-care. Did not eating enough earlier in the day precede the panic hunger? Experiment with adding more. Did you not give yourself enough break time? Consider adding a few more moments to briefly take deep breaths between meetings.

7 As uncomfortable as they are, panic hunger experiences will build the foundation to know how much self-care you need to add to your day. There's more on this in Chapter 7.

Remember, going through these experiences gives you important information on your body's specific needs. It is impossible to know this information without stumbling upon these uncomfortable experiences. Practice permission when they happen, consider the new data, and try to move on. Keep in mind everyone experiences panic hunger, so having these experiences is never a failure. It's just new data, and that is a win.

Am I emotionally hungry? What does it symbolize?

The last CHIP question gauges your current emotional hunger. If you check in and notice no physical hunger and still yearn to eat, this could be emotional hunger. Emotional hunger captures moments of yearning to eat without physical sensations. This type can be harder to pinpoint and riddled with shame when used as a cue to eat.

Someone once commented on my blog: "Learning the different types of hungers has been helpful yet I struggle most with eating when I am not hungry. Like I KNOW I am not hungry yet I eat the food anyway. Especially really tasty food. Or sometimes it isn't even that great and I am just watching TV after work then notice I have gone through a bag of chips. I don't remember tasting them!"

My favorite thing to wear while writing this book has been my Legalize Emotional Eating sweatshirt from Nicole Groman's online merchandise shop.[4] I get more nods, soft smiles, and whispered "thank yous" from strangers when I wear it. We all need a daily reminder for permission to eat emotionally. Especially emotionally.

Finding your Food Voice includes discerning the why behind eating without judgment. I want you to practice that same permission to feel and act on emotional hunger.

Let me be clear. Emotional eating is:

- normal
- healthy
- important
- a strength
- an effective coping mechanism.

Imagining your food thought superhighway again; all too often we have been conditioned to feel shame from eating outside of meal hunger. Why do we fear our normal response to feelings? This conditioning comes from cultural fear of weight gain tied to racism. This shame acts like bumpers blocking you from understanding what needs are being met with emotionally cued eating.

Can we pluck out the shame when noticing yearning to eat outside of hunger? I wish a set of tweezers was all we needed to repair this part of accessing your Food Voice. Practice at every CHIP looking for emotional hunger, normalizing it, and eating in response to the request if you want. Practice giving yourself compassion when you do.

"What about health?" you ask. I can hear some naysayers arguing against emotionally cued eating. My rebuttal remains that, across the globe and over time, people have always emotionally eaten. Even more, people always will. Food has always contained a mechanism for coping with anxiety, fear, happiness, and any other triggering emotion. It works with just one bite. Ignoring it or shaming yourself for using such a convenient, legal tool will only block you from your Food Voice.

Connecting with the symbolism behind emotionally cued eating will only help you better understand your body's physical and emotional needs. I find my clients experience less depression and improved health markers (like lower insulin, blood sugar, cholesterol, and blood pressure) as they rewrite their rules around emotional eating.

In Chapter 8 I will teach you more about repairing your emotionally cued eating part of your Food Voice. Until then, I encourage you to practice nonjudgmental curiosity. Instead of saying, "I shouldn't have eaten that. I wasn't even hungry!", try saying something like "I wonder what unspoken need eating is helping me meet." Using *should* to describe your eating pattern is maladaptive... meaning it won't get you anywhere but in a funk and dead end. Call out that *should* and step back to consider a bigger picture. Just like Rae and I discussed earlier in this book, try to stop *shoulding* on *yourself*.

After asking the questions

After going through the questions, take care of each unmet need as you can in the moment. There is no exact best way to do this, so practice giving yourself permission to try out different answers. Sometimes eating a slowly prepared meal will fit whereas other times the vending machine choice will satisfy. I expect at times food won't be what you reach for and that is okay. CHIPs allow for you to start the practice of taking care of your needs. Later in this book, you will learn ways to experiment with your nutrition to see what you and your body prefer.

If you find yourself confused on *what* to eat at each check-in, know there is no wrong choice. Practice identifying and responding to your unmet needs. Finding your Food Voice emerges when you *respond* to these needs rather than how you respond to them. If you feel blocked from making a decision, use these loose suggestions as a guide *only*. You will eventually outgrow them and make your own guiding principles.

Snack hunger

In the appendix, I made a list of food groups for you. Look through this list and place a checkmark next to the foods you enjoy and have access to consistently. Next time you identify a snack hunger, choose a food within at least one or two of these food groups. Serving sizes don't exist while finding your Food Voice. Practice having permission for smaller and larger amounts until you find your favorite stopping point.

Meal hunger

Just like snack hunger, use the food group list to satisfy mealtime needs. With a greater nourishment need, choose at least three or four food groups. Practice responding to meal hunger and notice the feedback, if any, you get from eating varying amounts. Do you like feeling a big umph after eating a meal? Or would you rather stop sooner and eat another meal again in a few hours? The choice is yours.

Eating amounts

If you find yourself having trouble knowing how much to eat, you are not doing it wrong. Neurodivergence, past trauma, and food insecurity have impacted my clients' ability to know how much to eat, and this may be the case for you, too. Working with a registered dietitian or health coach who is trained in how to help you find your Food Voice can help you build the directional blocks you need and give you support.

When determining how much to eat at a meal or snack, please know there is no correct answer. All food choices and amounts provide support. This includes even when you choose not to eat. I know you are trying to figure things out and it is okay to flail around to learn what you need. Try to focus on eating enough; this is the most important part of taking care of your food choices. Your body will get sluggish or tired, or you may get moody or a headache, when you have not eaten enough. You can also get more swirling thoughts about food. We all have days a few times a year where this happens. More dangerous signs of not eating enough include: lightheadedness, weakness, and dizziness. These are not normal, and I don't want you to ignore them. These are urgent signs that you need to be evaluated by a medical professional to be sure you are safe.

Pick your CHIP times

Most people need to eat at least every three to four hours. This helps keep your blood sugar at balanced levels to keep your brain supply of glucose adequate. If you had a lifetime without scripts and ample access to food, your brain would bring food thoughts to your awareness around every three to four hours. This awareness helps you prepare the food, make shopping lists, and eat enough. Keep in mind that every three to four hours is an *estimate only*: some folks need more than that, especially if they have experienced diets, eating disorder behaviors, or familial restrictive food rules.

You are going to select CHIP times. At these times, you will pause, compassionately ask yourself the barometer questions, and engage in self-care. For many people I have worked with, Paul included, these CHIPs were powerful tools to lessen food preoccupation and bring to the surface their Food Voice communication.

Let's pick times of day prearranged to be your CHIPs. I have found that setting up CHIPs every two to three hours helps prevent extreme hunger pangs. There's nothing wrong with those yet I appreciate how chaotic and urgent they can make the moment. More frequent check-in times will give you a calmer chance to decide how you feel hungry to eat, what hunger levels feel best for you to start eating, and even if you use hunger sensations at all to guide it.

Your first CHIP will be within an hour of waking up. Then, using your typical day as a guide, pick times every two to three hours to check in. You may have some parts of your day that are predetermined like a scheduled lunch break or dinner with your family. Use these *must break* times as guides and be sure you have CHIPs every two to three hours around them.

Most people I have worked with felt fine about their eating during a workday yet chaotic and overwhelmed in the evening. Scripts tend to get very loud when our day has more space. This is often a time of loneliness or other tough emotions. Your scripts take advantage of despair and carefully craft a distraction. CHIPs are vital in the evening because it will help rewire your brain for permission and compassion instead of rigid food and body thoughts. I will take you through how to move through these lonely times of day with compassion later in this chapter.

Something else to consider: I find most people desperately need to eat more often during the workday. Even though you may be busy during the day and feel okay with food, not eating as much during the day promotes that chaotic binge feeling at night. Eating more throughout the day tends to lessen that urgent extreme hunger, making food decisions easier and less rushed.

In case you are wondering, it usually takes about two weeks of CHIP practice to notice a difference in food thoughts. Be kind to yourself as you start this practice.

Ready to assign your CHIP times? Go to FindYourFoodVoiceBook.com or library.johnmurraylearning.com for a worksheet I have created for you. There you will find a place to record your times and a place to take note of how you answer CHIP questions. Do you have a complicated history with food journals? I always want food records to be optional, and if you can experiment with this different way it has tremendous power to get you out of the Diet Trap. Use your best judgment, though. You know yourself best and I trust you.

Are weekdays and weekends/days off from work drastically different? It's okay to make two different CHIP sequences based on whether you are working or not. Just be sure to start within an hour of waking up and check in every two to three hours.

What to do with food outside of your CHIPs

You have now set aside times throughout the day to reconnect with your mind and body. You know how to pause, ground, and go through a series of questions. Your CHIP to-do list is set. But what about the rest of the day?

Check-in props help you practice checking in *and* checking out. We have designed each CHIP to be thorough and frequent, yet you will still find your thoughts or cues centering around food and eating.

Paul wondered if it was okay to eat outside of CHIP times. "It sounds like these prompts are designed to keep me eating only at certain times. Is that correct?" he asked.

Please know this without a doubt from me: you have unconditional permission to eat whenever you want or need to eat. Check-in props are a tool to help you discern your Food Voice not another rigid tool to keep you from eating too much. Making another food rule will not help rather hinder your healing.

I told Paul to do three things when he noticed food thoughts or cravings outside of his CHIPs:

- Ground.
- Be curious.
- Experiment.

After grounding with a few deep breaths, be curious about what is going on. Some folks will even pull out their CHIP questions. Notice if you are getting a cue to eat, and try to name whether it is physical or emotional. Don't be surprised when judgment and shame come along with this information. Be wary of the *shoulds* like:

- I shouldn't have to eat since I ate X minutes ago.
- I shouldn't be hungry as it's not time.
- I shouldn't deal with my boredom, stress [insert any other emotion] via eating.

When you notice these *shoulds* via thoughts or feelings, remind yourself the three core qualities to your Food Voice:

- flexible
- nurturing
- kind.

Practice noticing how the *shoulds* do not match these three qualities. Imagine the *shoulds* floating down a river away from the moment and stay grounded where you are. Resist the urge to swim in that river with the *shoulds*; instead, practice naming them and letting them move on.

Do I recommend eating in these moments? That is not my question to answer because there is no right or wrong. These moments are morally neutral. I recommend you allow these moments to just be data-collecting experiments. Many times you will eat, and many times you will not. These choices will impact your next CHIP time and give you even more insight into your Food Voice. More insight points you in the direction of healing and growth.

Paul worked hard on letting go of the *shoulds* outside of his CHIPs. He went with the idea to experiment with gusto. Paul found that, when he was physically hungry outside of his CHIP times and didn't eat, he hit panic hunger soon thereafter. He really did not like getting to that vulnerable place. Even though he learned he couldn't always avoid panic hunger—he is human, after all—he considered eating enough at his CHIPs at least to be a minimum to experience a lot less panicky food dilemmas.

Emotional hunger was not so linear. Paul found eating for stress relief at times helped him better focus whereas other times it made him sluggish. This lack of consistency drove him bananas and it may do that for you, too.

I-Should-Eat scripts have taught us rigid routines are safe. In a way, these specifics are a set of mismatched boundaries clearing our head because they remind us we are being good. Emotional eating especially outside of your CHIPs may feel wrong, yet know that is just a part of your downloaded scripts. You are not doing anything wrong when you are taking care of your needs—whether physical or emotional.

I want to remind you as many times as I can: you have unconditional permission to eat anytime anywhere with what is accessible to you. Choosing to eat or not eat does not determine your worth or goodness. Being a human already gives you all of that.

Here's the work for you to do: discern when you want to emotionally eat and when you want to pick another tool to meet your emotional needs. Over the next two weeks, practice your CHIP routine. Notice when you emotionally eat during your CHIPs and outside of them. Begin to notice how they impact, if at all, your energy levels, emotions, focus, and mood. This takes a tremendous amount of bandwidth, yet I promise it won't always be this strenuous. Like learning to ride a bike or type, eventually this will become something you don't have to think about so intensely.

Be wary of the one thing that will block your CHIPs routine: your past *I-Should-Eat* scripts. When they pop up, and they will, announce their arrival. Let the scripts know you have been waiting for them. Tell them they are no longer needed and watch from the riverbanks as they float away. The more scripts you send off while emotionally eating, the more connection and repair will happen for you and your Food Voice.

Keep this reminder close by: your Food Voice is not about keeping you from eating too much; it's about taking care of yourself including eating enough.

Will you always require your CHIPs?

As you go off and practice these new guardrails, keep in mind it will take time and practice to repair your Food Voice communication. I am unsure how long you will need your CHIPs. This depends on how complicated your eating history is and the oppressive systems you encounter. Many of my clients over the years needed just a month with CHIPs to reconnect with their Food Voice whereas others still like using CHIPs years later. You will probably fall somewhere in between.

Taking your pivot step is hard work and good work. Be proud of what you have repaired already. I would love to read about your *ahas* happening in real time. Tag me on social media using @FoodVoiceRD and use the hashtag #FindMyFoodVoice.

Dear a girl who needs help,

I wish the world didn't interfere with how you take care of your eating. Please be compassionate with yourself as you uncover the depth of your diet wound. Remind yourself often how you did nothing wrong. You were never the problem. No matter how you coped, you survived and that is your strength. You are not addicted to food, rather clinging to your humanity. Consider adding guardrails to tap you on the shoulder and bring your awareness to the present. Ask yourself what unmet needs you have. Practice lovingly embracing those needs even when it feels impossible. This will be hard work yet will add up to repair your complicated eating history.

Love,
Food

Dear Food letter activity

Write a letter to Food describing what comes up for you when you consider not relying on the scale as a measure of progress or worth. What comes up for you when you consider not relying on your scripts anymore? Let yourself brainstorm all the emotions and thoughts that come up with these next steps. Communicate them all to Food to help you hold on to them.

Voice Finder Cord activity

Hold the green family of strings. Measure one finger width from the last knot. While you are doing this, practice grounding your mind and body. Make six knots in total, separating all of them about one finger width apart. These six knots represent the six questions to ask during your CHIPs:

- Am I hot or cold?
- What am I feeling? Or, if this fits better, what messages am I getting from my brain?
- Do I need to use the bathroom?
- What are my thoughts focused on?
- Am I physically hungry? How do I know?
- Am I emotionally hungry? What does it symbolize?

References

1 Bremner, J. D., Campanella, C., Khan, Z., Shah, M., Hammadah, M., Wilmot, K., et al. (2018). Brain correlates of mental stress-induced myocardial ischemia. *Psychosomatic Medicine* 80(6), 515–25; Jacob, L. (2018). Post-traumatic stress symptoms are associated with physical multimorbidity: findings from the Adult Psychiatric Morbidity Survey 2007. *Journal of Affective Disorders* 232, 385–92.
2 Fairburn, C. G. (2013). *Overcoming Binge Eating: The Proven Program to Learn Why You Binge and How You Can Stop*. The Guilford Press.
3 https://www.apa.org/monitor/2023/04/sensations-eating-disorders-suicidal-behavior (accessed November 27, 2023).
4 https://www.nicolegroman.com/product-page/legalize-emotional-eating-sweatshirt.

6

Release

Dear Food,

I realized we had a complicated relationship after reading *Intuitive Eating* for the first time. I wanted to teach myself the "right" way to eat. I thought I was doing well and generally feeling at peace. Until it was pointed out I was following the "intuitive eating" diet, and this launched a pretty steep decline in my recovery. Was everything I had learned the last three years completely wrong? I do not feel like I have it in me to stay on this path, and I continue to be in a half-recovered space. Working through my disordered food behaviors illuminated how I have a lot of personal trauma and feelings which I was using disordered behaviors to cover up. As I work through those, I notice the disordered food behaviors creeping back in like old friends.

Diet culture is everywhere. And because it is everywhere, I feel exhausted by constantly defending my position to people and not giving in to the allure of what I know now to be another diet.

Yoga has been a refuge, but I attended a yoga teacher training informational session and left feeling completely defeated after learning that one of the training modules was around "how to eat like a yogi". My extended family gatherings that involve food consist of comments about amounts of food, "good/bad" food, and needing to "work off" the food. Sharing my own baked treats with coworkers inevitably invites a litany of body and diet comments as well as their own personal justifications for eating or not eating. I created an Instagram account for my dog because I thought it would be fun. Do you know how much diet culture permeates Instagrams about dogs? I cannot shut off the continuous diet culture.

Perhaps I am not fully on board with intuitive eating and Health at Every Size (HAES) and there are still pieces of diet culture I am hanging on to. All I know right now, Food, is I am angry. I am angry that I know my food behaviors aren't healthy but I want to keep doing them because it feels like I am in control. I have so much shame for having this problem at all that I can hardly admit it to myself.

Will I ever feel normal around you, Food?

Will I ever want to take care of my body instead of punishing myself? Can I enjoy you, Food, without feeling an intense desire to exercise or restrict you later? Can I trust you, Food, knowing that my IBS may cause intense intestinal pain and fear of you, Food? Will I be able to go to my doctor and not be completely obsessed for weeks after accidentally seeing my weight (and shame for feeling good that it was lower than what I thought)? It all feels too much, and I feel entirely ungrounded. I realize this letter is even contradictory, stating I wish I could have my old food behaviors back and also knowing I have learned and made progress. I am just not sure, Food, that I am on the right path, or even what the right path is.

Sincerely,
Wanting to Check Out

I hope you are proud of your work so far pivoting away from routine rigid food thoughts. Do you feel a bit freer? I call this first taste of freedom the "non-diet honeymoon."

Matilda met with me during her non-diet honeymoon. She had picked her CHIPs at the last week's appointment and we met to see if she needed to fine-tune them. Instead of making adjustments, Matilda thought everything was perfect. She was also experiencing new emotions around her foodways. "For the first time in years I ordered what I wanted at brunch with friends. I feel so free around food!"

I told her I was happy she felt something around food she hadn't in a long time. Celebrate this win *and* know this may be a pause before the storm. I added, "Please know that, if the excitement fades and things get scary again, that doesn't mean you are doing anything wrong. It just means we still live in a diet culture."

When you first start tiptoeing away from rigid eating plans, you, like Matilda, might feel a sense of relief and newfound excitement. I appreciate years have passed without permission to eat however you want, whenever you want, without rules. While this type of freedom is your human birthright, eating chips out of the bag or having a boozy brunch probably feels like the ultimate rebellion.

When I first started helping clients find their Food Voice, I didn't see the pattern I see now. Not everyone experiences a non-diet honeymoon yet, when they do, the crash afterwards can stop healing in its tracks.

A non-diet honeymoon takes place when the drastic side of diets meets raw permission to eat. Just like the pendulum discussed in Chapter 5, picture this pendulum swinging from a mean dictator yelling food rules to a smiling crush inviting you to a carefree meal filled with laughter. Often your CHIPs help push the pendulum away from the food rules and toward those long-yearned-for blissful moments with food. Your brain will feel a buzz as it finally has a break from constant food negativity.

This feels good, so enjoy it. As I told Matilda, just know the feeling may be fleeting. It is a pendulum, after all, and living with the diet industry's control means that something will eventually remind you of why the rules were there in the first place.

Your brain may very well get pulled violently back toward an *I-Should-Eat* script. As it fixates back on the negative and seeks order with food, please do not think you are failing. You are truly surviving and making your way to understand what you need to be thriving.

From honeymoon to release

Finding your Food Voice includes steps that don't feel good. One of the steps is what comes crumbling down after a non-diet honeymoon. While you probably have experienced a complicated history with food for years, I predict this will feel different.

Why? Going back to the pendulum, remember your food thoughts were used to a constant tug of war. With your first few days or weeks within your CHIPs, you may experience an exhilarating feeling you haven't experienced before with eating. Unfortunately, there is something else around the corner. Newton's Third Law states that for every action there is an equal and opposite reaction—and this holds true when mending your Food Voice.

When Matilda came back in a few weeks later, I could feel the energy shift as soon as she walked in the door. A few days earlier someone said something about her body that tipped her scripts into full blast mode. "I feel exhausted. My brain keeps saying this feeling is too much, but I keep hearing you say in my head 'Feelings don't last forever, and they can't hurt you.' I am repeating that at every CHIP. I am grateful you gave me the heads-up this would happen, but when will it get easier?"

Your scripts know that you finding your Food Voice will end them. I often picture them getting angrily fired up when folks reject them so efficiently and joyfully the first few times. The scripts use this as rocket fuel to bring up every past bad body thought and food punishment. If you are reading this before your non-diet honeymoon, name it as such when it happens. When the pendulum swings back toward the scripts, name that too. Maybe throw in a few powerful "fuck offs" to let them know you are on to them and one step ahead and ready to *release* them.

Gently remind yourself that scripts are predictable assholes, only trying to disconnect you from yourself, disarm you of your intuition, and distract you from the oppressive systems provoking all the pain. The more you can step back and notice what is happening within the pendulum, the more insight you will gain into your Food Voice. This skill will help you with the intense steps ahead. You can do this, and I am rooting for you.

Are you ready to release?

I encourage you to practice your CHIPs for two weeks or more as you connect with this chapter's concept of Release.* This chapter explores the range of emotions that predictably come up as you practice your CHIPs. Many of these experiences have kept previous clients of mine stuck or disheartened. It may feel like you are doing it wrongly. You are not.

---

* Not ready to do the CHIPs and wondering if you should keep reading? Ouch, I just wrote *should*! Yes, keep reading. Getting an advanced notification of complex emotions will only help you.

Feeling free for the first time since kindergarten, Rae almost skipped into my office after our first scheduled meeting following their CHIP design session. "I think you cured me! I almost blew off the CHIP plan because it didn't sound like it would do anything but WHOA! What a difference! We may not need another session for a while."

While I love seeing clients happy, I had heard this hopeful decree many times before. Having a plan forward ignites a fire that has been absent. Unfortunately, this first fire is only kindling and tends to burn out soon thereafter.

We aren't meant to be on fire all of the time. Diets like to promise they can deliver and shoot spark after spark to keep us believing in them. Unfortunately, your first steps away from your scripts may fall into the worn-in magical thinking grooves carved out without your consent by diet culture.

Unlike diets that keep spewing lies, finding your Food Voice is grounded in reality. Hope is fleeting and it will be now, too. And that doesn't mean you are doing it incorrectly. In fact, the next few uncomfortable emotional phases I witness after the CHIP guardrails confirm progress, not regression.

At their next appointment, Rae had confused tears sitting on my office's green couch. "I was relieved as my CHIPs allowed more space for me to not think about food. I didn't think they could do anything but they did. And I was excited—exhilarated even—like I was in love. I was walking on cloud nine thinking all of my food and body struggles were over. Then ..."

I tried to meet Rae's gaze. They met mine, and Rae took a deep breath. "I think I am doing it wrong now."

"Why's that, Rae?"

Then Rae said something many people had said before them:

"I feel so ... sad."

Breaking up with diets and reconnecting with the possibilities of body liberation feels amazing at first. You will feel a buzz and elation. And of course you will—because after all these years trapped in diet industry lies, you will feel a weight lifted.

It may also feel a lot like that familiar hopeful buzz a new diet brings. Only now, moving away from diets doesn't keep pushing you towards the narrative of toxic positivity. Rejecting diets and repairing your Food

Voice is hard work for many reasons, especially because the world hasn't even recognized that diet culture is a problem.

I told Rae, "Sometimes finding your Food Voice is sad. There is no avoiding it, and experiencing this sadness tends to be the next step for most of my clients. We can push pause here and take it slow or we can go through it. The choice is yours, Rae."

They chose to go through. Will you?

Common emotions at this stage: sadness and grief

Rae shared with me the details surrounding their sadness. And, wow, was it loaded.

Rae let me know they didn't anticipate how different normal conversations would be while finding their Food Voice. Rae said, "I feel even more different now because I cannot join conversations about new diets or weight-loss goals. I am sad to not have that easy connection with people."

I told Rae, "This is a tough spot while finding their Food Voice. Dieting is normal eating these days. Connections are made over meal planning, fad diets, and boot camps. You may find giving up diets will make some relationships shift or feel strange."

I encourage you to surround yourself with as many non-dieting, normal eaters as possible. If you can't find them in real life, consider joining a support group whether live or virtually. Work with a counselor, dietitian, or health coach to help you make these steps. Just be sure they ascribe to a weight-inclusive approach and are trained not to focus on weight loss.

Next, Rae mentioned how reality hit them one day: diets really are never going to work for them. Like *really*. Rae was surprised how this moment felt like a punch to the gut. All the hopeful fantasies were rushing away from them: the promise of a better life with more options and safety. Rae said, "I am so done with the roller coaster diets bring to my life, but now that the dust has settled, I feel more hopelessness. It really was all a lie."

Eating according to your own body's messages may feel odd, novel, or strange. It may sound exciting and scary. Soon after the excitement, most people I speak with grieve. They grieve for all the years wasted on dieting and the seductive fantasy diets had in their life. Moving past this space can take time, so I invite you to take all the time you need.

I told Rae connecting with the sadness and grief will feel uncomfortable yet is the only way to get to your Food Voice. When I notice clients connecting to this tough space, I know they are connecting with their truth and are repairing. It just doesn't feel good. Please keep in mind that this does not mean you are doing it wrongly. The diet industry is the one doing it wrongly.

Common emotions at this stage: anger and resentment

After I had this session on sadness and grief with Rae, I next started to look for anger. Everyone has their own unique path to finding their Food Voice, and most will have patterns and themes. When the session concluded, I told Rae to notice anything else that came up alongside their sadness. They were not delighted there was more around the corner!

I told Rae what I offer now to you: I am here with you as you navigate all of this. The feelings will not hurt you, but diets will.

I knew that Rae was starting to appreciate the shame they were holding on to because diets didn't work for them. It wasn't their fault, and it's not your fault. Diets are a shitty tool. You've been manipulated by big oppressive systems and massive, rich corporations to believe you are to blame.

The way I picture it: you've been successfully manipulated so you are wearing a very heavy shame cloak. Bingeing and food addiction experiences connect to the diet industry's manufactured shame and lack of permission for pleasure. Doing all this work to connect to your authentic Food Voice probably has you appreciating that you haven't been falling off the wagon all these years and that it is time to burn that wagon down.

I knew Rae was connecting the dots that systems had told them to feel this shame and blame and realizing this was misplaced. Connecting with who is to blame usually brings on a flood of anger. Ouch, it can hurt and be uncomfortable, especially if you don't have permission to feel anger just like Rae.

This pissed-off rage is a vital stop while finding your Food Voice because it will fuel you for the next portion of your journey. It gives you the direction and places the blame where it belongs: away from you and on to cultural systems like racism, weight stigma, sexism, homophobia, xenophobia, and so forth. And wow, is that heavy!

While I root for you like Rocky Balboa's coach, I appreciate that I am in the easy part of the ring, safely behind the ropes. I also have experience witnessing others so I can see a bit ahead. Know that this place may feel scary and exhilarating. It won't feel like you are connecting with hunger or fullness because releasing the feelings of sadness, grief, anger, and resentment takes up so much space. You may literally feel as though you are so full of anger that hunger cues will be miles away.

Do you wonder how long these emotions will be in this space while finding their Food Voice? The anger is draining! There is no way to answer how long it takes because it is individual to you. It depends on your lived experiences, your support systems, and the systems you must navigate to live your life. I hope you give yourself compassion and patience while navigating this part of the journey.

Your relationship with anger

Traci was a multiracial teen recovering from an eating disorder. You met her mother, Keisha, in Chapter 2 as she was starting the process to access eating disorder treatment for Traci yet struggled to get her a diagnosis. Traci sat on my green couch as she had weekly over the past year strategizing with me on how to meet her nutrition needs while regaining access to her Food Voice. The last few weeks, I could tell her brain was finally able to access emotions and she was starting to be herself again.

One day, she mentioned to me how angry she felt. She was connecting to all the time she wasted worrying about each calorie she ate and whether she was eating too much. She realized this impacted her experience of high school: she didn't join clubs because they served pizza at the meetings and ate her lunch by herself because it was too hard to eat in front of others. As her brain was now getting enough nutrition, she realized how much she had missed. And she was pissed.

Traci said, "I feel so *mad*. I was robbed of my middle school and first two years of high school. I missed all the fun and have no friends. This eating disorder has taken so much from me. I don't think I have ever felt this angry and know it was because I was starving so I couldn't feel anything. But now I really do! I feel everything! And I hate this angry feeling. I feel like I am always killing the vibe."

Somehow our discussion evolved into addressing how racist and sexist belief systems lead us to believe our anger disrupts the status quo and that we need to disengage from this anger to keep the peace. These systems taught Traci her feelings were not important.

I told Traci, "An angry feminist makes the world uncomfortable. But that is not the feminist's problem—it is the world's."

"Oh, no," Traci recoiled, "I am definitely not a feminist—they are bitchy all of the time and can't take a joke. They just want to make everyone uncomfortable."

I said, "But there is a lot to be angry about. You have been starving yourself for five years just to keep the peace. You are valid. Your feelings are valid. They are showing us how wrong this world is, and I wish more people told you that expressing these feelings *helps* the world rather than harms it. I am sorry you've been told to hold back in order to keep the world from noticing the problems."

Traci stared blankly for a few moments. Twice, she opened her mouth and closed it without saying a word. She looked around the room then at her hands. Eventually she took a deep breath and let it out. With that she looked over at me with tears in her eyes and said with resolve, "I think I am getting it."

Over the next few months, I noticed Traci slowly unpacked the complexity of her anger. And you can, too. So much began when Traci acknowledged the oppressive systems tricking her into believing that she was only acceptable when she was playing the cool girl. From there, she connected with a therapist with similar identities to Traci's. Together, they formed Traci's version of intersectional feminism that helped her feel powerful and aligned with her Food Voice. Traci told me this type of feminism gave permission for anger and acknowledged it was okay when she couldn't express it.

If you, like Traci, at times feel unsafe about releasing anger, please know you are not doing it wrongly. Remind yourself this world is unjust, and those with more privilege have work to do. If you live with identities that give you more space to release challenging emotions like anger, let's work together to make safer spaces for Black, Brown, Indigenous, and other people of color to explore and release. Just another reminder that finding your Food Voice, and unpacking all its complicated bits, will not only help you yet also help people like Traci find theirs.

When these uncomfortable emotions hit

Anger consistently shows up for folks while finding their Food Voice. So much so that I think it is important to give you a heads-up that it will be coming so you can prepare for its intensity and consider repairing your own relationship with anger.

My personal instinctive learned response to anger is to shrink, hide, cover up, and hold it in. My gut reaction isn't to yell, beat my fists, or even express anger, but rather to pretend it is not there. Cool as a cucumber on the outside while bursting at the seams inside. I want to minimize the discomfort in the hope that, by ignoring it, this unwelcomed emotion will buzz off.

Can you relate to this? What is your reaction to anger (or frustration, overwhelm, agitation, or other similar emotions)? Is it like mine, or different? *How* is it different?

Getting a graduate degree in mental health counseling, decades of individual therapy, and eons of introspective work helps me to unravel these instincts and notice the anger. Sometimes I can express it, albeit not always in the way I hope. Tolerating natural, normal, healthy anger is a part of my life work, and I have noticed it is for many with a complicated history with food.

How we relate to food often mirrors how we relate to anger. This often sounds like one or more of these:

- Minimizing anger while holding on to a false truth that you don't need to eat that much; minimizing your need to eat just like minimizing your normal anger.
- Choosing not to eat because you don't want anyone to hear you open up a noisy chip bag or the clanging of a utensil on a plate; hiding your need to eat just like you can hide your normal anger.
- Making sure to take the empty food containers to the trash or even move them to a trash can away from your home after eating certain

forbidden foods; hiding your needs because you don't want to be too much of a burden.

- Waiting to eat until you are alone even if panic hunger hits; not allowing yourself to meet basic needs because of the false belief that it is immoral to have these needs just like the very presence of anger establishes you as a bad person. No one is allowed to see or know this.

How has your relationship with anger mirrored your relationship with food?

Releasing while finding your Food Voice encourages you to notice anger and related emotions. Name them and normalize them. It includes recognizing the healthy human need to express, rather than hold in, anger even if you can't quite do that yet. Be gentle with yourself as you notice the discomfort and try when you can to lean into it. Remember feelings—all of them—cannot hurt you. Recognize any blocks or hurdles life has thrown at you to keep you from expressing your full range of anger-related emotions.

Pivoting away from our learned responses to anger helps us move the needle away from the instinctual shame blocking our Food Voice. Point the blame instead to where it belongs: oppressive systems like the diet industry, ableism, healthism, transphobia, xenophobia, and all the rest rooted in racism.

Release the anger. Break some dishes. Scream and sob at the top of your lungs. Reject the shame downloaded into your brain without your consent: your anger is normal and healthy. It is vital. It literally feeds you and the earth. Releasing it will not only help you find your Food Voice but also help the rest of us connect with our own.

Once you release these first layers of emotions related to anger, more feelings will be nestled there waiting. Your anger release may feel like ripping off a Band-Aid to show you the wound you didn't know was there underneath. It may sting from the years of punishing scripts, overexercise, and body shame. What comes up for you after releasing anger? Many people describe intense grief. When you can tolerate it, I encourage you to notice what the grief is telling you and try not to minimize it.

Like anger, we live in a culture where grief isn't accepted. We are expected to acknowledge change and move on. Many of us have been programmed to act as if grief doesn't even exist. Why is that? Traci told me she didn't want to share her grief with her mom because she didn't want to be a burden. Traci acknowledged how hard her mom worked to advocate for her and now Keisha finally seemed less stressed. Traci said she would feel ungrateful expressing this grief to her mom.

None of us want to feel like a burden. Opening up our grief and sharing it takes up uncomfortable space and can feel too much. We have been trained to just shut off our connections to grief. Unfortunately, these societal rules will keep us stuck. Exploring the grief anger has released will help you repair your Food Voice.

Consider these options as starting points to allow grief's tension to lessen its grip and help you move forward:

- Grab your journal or open your phone's notes app and do a brain dump. Try not to judge, and allow your brain to let it all out without regard for grammar or logic. Note the different ways and places grief is showing up in your body.
- Is your grief localized to a certain part of your body? Practice self-compassion as you connect these dots and take breaks when you need them.
- Give yourself permission to explore your script grief with a therapist, coach, dietitian, or a supportive friend. Unpack stuck points as many times as you need because grief has no distinct timeline.
- Consider adding community while grieving. Other people finding their Food Voice also grieve the years spent hating their body and are trying to find new ways to live. I highly recommend Bri Campos's work within her Body Grievers podcast and community—https://bodyimagewithbri.com/
- Does your culture have any grief traditions? Even if your family of origin didn't teach you how to express grief, your ancestors may have had a way. What can you take from your inherited death rituals to help you process what you are going through now?
- Take your time. There is no rush. Taking breaks and centering self-care is not avoiding grief, but rather tending to it.

When feeling is too much

My graduate degree provided tools I had been searching for as an early-career dietitian. A semester on empathy, another on multicultural counseling, and the daily curious conversations fed me. It also drained me. I remember after a particularly emotionally tough day at my second-year counseling internship—which happened to be at a children's hospice—I found myself in a fit of solo anger taking a tennis racket to my bed. I did this for a good ten minutes then collapsed on the floor sobbing.

Nothing like the concept of death combined with child psychology to really get me to this raw place. It was at this intense moment I realized I needed a break. I had a decision to make during this time in school: continue on to pursue another semester to help me maintain counseling licensure or finish in a few months. In the back of my mind, I was also considering a PhD. Sitting on the floor exhausted after this particular sob, I knew graduate school was over for me. I needed more time to take care of myself. I decided to finish the semester, graduate without any bonus academic hours, and take care of me.

What did I logistically need? I needed to check out. I remember telling my peers, "I just need not to be self-aware for a little while. If I continue on in academia, it will be a waste because I will be checked out. I don't want it that much."

Everyone encouraged me to do what I needed to do, yet I always wonder whether there was some judgment because I wouldn't keep going. Did I lack perseverance? If I just pushed through, would I be Dr. Duffy Dillon right now?

Maybe, but I knew I needed a break. I do wonder whether, if I had found ways to disconnect more often, I would have chosen a different direction. I also know that watching reality TV and reading *People* magazine after graduation provided more health and wellbeing than I had experienced in two years!

Matilda came into my office and sat down on my green couch looking exhausted. She had been doing her CHIPs for over a month and bravely naming the feelings coming up. Anger, overwhelm, fear, frustration, and disappointment all came through now that she had cleared space in her head for them. At this particular session, though, her exhaustion painted a different picture:

"This feels intense all of the time. I am feeling the feelings and ashamed I can't take it all. I need a break but know that is wrong."

I gasped a little under my breath, and I remember thinking I hoped she hadn't noticed. My breath tripped up because Matilda was sifting through these tough emotions and believed that this was the only way forward: a constant whipping post for whatever came up.

"Can we focus in on that shame for a moment?" I asked. She nodded and I replied, "You are not doing anything wrong. You are brave and tired. It sounds like you need a disconnection break; maybe even some good ol' dissociation."

Our psyches benefit from grounded self-awareness yet they can take only so much before we need to check out. That seems obvious to me now after working with folks like Matilda and others with a complicated food history. I appreciate we are not taught this, myself included. I needed a tennis racket and a big sob; I wonder what sign will tell you that you need to disconnect?

If you are harmed by many different oppressive systems, I expect this to happen sooner rather than later while you are finding your Food Voice. Please give yourself permission to not always do your CHIPs or name your feelings. It's okay when the big feelings become intolerable and you need to self-soothe. I encourage you to gather a list of things that help you disconnect or even dissociate as you process the probable traumas that are provoking these intense emotions.

To get you started, here are some things my clients and I have found to be easily accessed when needing a break:

- Watch your comfort show on television.
- Color.
- Craft.
- Call or text a friend.
- Scroll social media.
- Read easy-to-read, pleasurable materials—magazines, books, etc.
- Stare out the window.
- Paint your nails.
- Fidget.
- Play video games.
- Emotionally eat—yes, I mean it.

Emotional eating may not be as powerful while releasing

Paul walked into my office for a follow-up appointment visibly angry. He had been consistently trying to eat enough to avoid panic hunger via his CHIPs the last few weeks and he had been hopeful and calm at recent appointments. This appointment, though, he sat on the green couch and glared at me. I squinted and gave him a few moments to speak first.

"Were your ears burning this weekend? Because I was mad at you."

Paul went on to fill me in on a particularly tough workweek and losing a case. He tried to keep up with his CHIPs and did manage to eat throughout the day most of these days, which I saw as a big win. Once Friday came, a surge of emotions plus exhaustion hit him like a ton of bricks.

On the way home from work Friday night, Paul stopped at a few fast-food restaurants. "I knew I needed to be comforted, and that was going to be the only thing that hit the right nerve to help me sleep."

I was on the edge of my seat wondering what happened next, but Paul didn't say anything for at least a minute as a flood of feelings showed across his face.

Eventually, he restarted. "I tried to emotionally eat yet it did nothing. It didn't soothe or calm me down. It was literally just food. It had no power. So I was sitting in my car with all this food and all the feelings I'd tucked away all week. I wanted... no, I *needed* to numb out. And the food did nothing." He broke down.

I watched as Paul sobbed. He tried to keep going, yet his hiccupping breaths took precedence over verbal communication. In this moment, I knew Paul was releasing more emotions than can be named and he was tolerating them. I also saw how much he needed a check-out moment yet felt unprepared.

As Paul's breathing evened back out, I asked permission to explore what was happening that Friday night in his car. I had some guesses.

I explained to Paul that he was doing amazing self-care knowing he needed a disconnecting break. Reaching for emotional eating in those moments makes sense. What also makes sense is that, as your awareness deepens, that emotional eating will not provide the same comfort.

What Paul experienced—emotional eating no longer buffering from reality—commonly happens while finding your Food Voice. There have been hundreds of office sobs on the green couch yet the most surprising tears come from clients who no longer find comfort in emotional eating.

Just like Paul, if this happens to you, you may experience a new low or sense of desperation. Remember, feelings cannot hurt you and yet the scripts will.

I encourage you to practice other techniques to self-soothe along with emotional eating. Experiment with many ways to disconnect or dissociate. Will these options feel just as good? Will they be just as effective? Probably not, especially in the beginning. Practicing these alternatives will eventually give them more power. At the same time, you will be practicing your CHIPs and getting better at feeling your feelings. You will begin to tolerate more discomfort and trust that feelings come and go.

Rae experienced this shift in emotional eating power, too. Rae emailed me between sessions to let me know how intolerable the emotions became when emotional eating didn't calm them down. At our next session, after Rae bravely recognized they did indeed tolerate those tough moments, we strategized for next time.

Keep in mind that, with every twist and turn while you find your Food Voice, you are given data to help you with the next leg of the journey. You make a stumble? Consider what you wish you had done differently. You've checked out and feel ashamed? Consider the need to take a break. You've said, "Fuck it!" and restricted something? Remind yourself you are living in a sea of *I-Should-Eat* scripts singing their siren call. Sometimes we fall.

When Rae and I strategized for next time, we ended up creating something we named their Food Voice Toolkit. Rae wanted an accessible resource to use when they were triggered to diet that would guide them toward compassion and curiosity rather than shame and blame. Creating it when grounded in our session helped Rae gather the tools they needed in tough moments.

Here's what we included:

- Voice Finder Cord.
- Sayings, quotes, and mantras that redirect toward one's Food Voice and away from *I-Should-Eat* scripts. Some client favorites include:

- o It's okay to not be okay.
- o Feelings can't hurt me.
- o Feelings are impermanent.
- o I am worthy just as I am.
- o I don't need to be fixed but the world does.
- o I am more than my feelings.
- o It's okay to be angry.
- o It's okay to eat emotionally.
- o It's okay to binge.
- o Each bite of food can't kill or cure me. Don't give food too much power.

- Life will deliver more powerful statements on a silver platter; write them down and place them in your Food Voice Toolkit.
- Phone numbers of friends, family, or other supportive people who you know you can connect with in the messy places.
- Fidgets or other manipulatives to help you release anxiety.
- Your favorite Spotify playlist name. Check out the Find Your Food Voice Playlist if you need another at FindYourFoodVoiceBook.com or library.johnmurraylearning.com.
- Scents that ground you or help you disconnect. Clients have put in candles, essential oils, or perfumes that remind them of someone or something supportive.
- Shelf-stable food that satisfies and can be a tool you need in the moment—whether to energize or disconnect. Many clients will wrap a note around the food giving your future self sweet reminders that it is important self-care to soothe and how brave they are being.

At the following session, Rae brought in an ornately carved wooden box filled with all of the items we named in our previous meeting. Their Food Voice Toolkit was special. In that moment I knew every Food Voice Toolkit needs to be unique to the owner and cherished. Just like your own Food Voice, your box will hold things most dear to you on your journey ahead. I encourage you to make yours special: taking care of your wounds and the feelings that come from them deserves a unique home that feels like support just by looking at it.

Finding your Food Voice sometimes involves tough-to-tolerate emotions. Release the notion that any are wrong, or worse, that you are doing it incorrectly. You are exactly where you are supposed to be.

While in this spot of your journey it may be tough to see how far you have come; one day soon, you will recognize how brave you are. You are especially brave right now. I am proud of you and rooting for you.

When you opened this book, you may not have thought it was possible that you could rewrite your complicated history with food. But you have stuck with it, read each page, and completed every exercise. The rest of the journey will help you mend the biggest wounds and strengthen your connection with your Food Voice.

Dear Wanting to Check Out,

We know you feel scammed out of healing. It's not your fault intuitive eating became another diet industry tool. Even more, you have a lot to be angry about. We appreciate this anger makes things more unclear and keeps you guessing about what to do next. We believe you can mend your complicated history with us and your body by allowing your Food Voice to emerge in the way you need it. When you can, pause and feel. What emotions and messages are coming up for you? None are wrong. All give you information. Consider the way you learned intuitive eating and other non-diet tools filtered through oppressive systems–how would healing look if we didn't have this muck? What if you instead had permission to feel it all and eat whatever you want when you want? We trust you to take care of you and rooting for you to trust yourself too.

Love,
Food

Dear Food letter activity

Write a letter to Food about what you need to release while pivoting away from your scripts. Be sure to include how your relationship with anger and related emotions may keep some stuck too long.

Voice Finder Cord activity

Hold the purple string family. Consider which emotions, experiences, and messages you want to release. Some you will know instantly on reading this whereas others will emerge over time while finding your Food Voice. Make a knot representing all of those known and those still left unspoken. Honor their meaning, then picture them all being gently carried away down a river.

After braiding about an inch or two, secure with a knot. Trim your cord to leave as much as you like after this last knot.

7

Practice

Dear Food,

We have had a difficult relationship for a very long time. I am in the middle of working hard to be successful in my college career and other life goals, but I can't ignore my fear of and addiction to you that have always followed me like a creeping shadow. I was unhappy with my body from an early age; I recall looking back in my diary and complaining about my size (I was at a smaller weight at that time) when I was seven; even back then I attributed my problems to you. Puberty hit me like a truck and I grew too quickly, gaining stretch marks all over my thighs, hips, and breasts. I blamed you for that, too.

As a teen, I gradually started putting on weight and suffering from mysterious little things that I just thought were a part of being a growing woman. My periods were irregular and heavy; I had borderline high cholesterol and was diagnosed with prediabetes in high school. I had such low energy and craved a nap every single day. I suffered from terrible panic disorder and depression, and was put on medication that I've continued to take for almost six years now. My acne was so bad that it made my skin itchy and red, and I spent over eight years trying at least ten different topical and medicinal treatments. Eventually, my dermatologist's assistant (a woman) suggested I had PCOS. I did the blood work and consulted with my gynecologist; it turned out they were right.

I was immediately put on birth control to manage my periods, with a promise that none of these medications would affect my steadily rising weight. I sought out the help of my GP multiple times for my weight gain and other symptoms. But she just agreed to whatever I suggested, whether it be medications, diets, or somewhat suspicious natural treatments.

Needless to say, Food, none of it worked. I restricted my consumption of you to only about X calories a day. I tried X diet. I hit the gym hard X times a week, following the instructions of other women online who said they had "cured" their PCOS. I tried quitting birth control even if it meant painful periods.

My weight has stayed the highest it's been. I am miserable at parties; seeing my skinny friends eat pizza and chips makes me so upset I want to peel myself out of my own skin. If I enjoy even a little bit of you, I feel immediately riddled with guilt and shame.

I have finally admitted to myself that none of these diets is working, and it isn't my fault or necessarily yours either, Food. The thing is, though, even though part of me knows this is true, I still hate my body, and I hate what you do to it. And I hate that I hate the way I am.

Will our relationship ever improve? Will I ever find the right combination of you that benefits my body the most? Will I be able to realize the difference between dieting or a final lifestyle change? And lastly, will I ever be happy with you around?

Sincerely,
Struggling for Life

"I am ready for gentle nutrition," Elena (she/her) directed me before I had even sat down to start our session. I had been hired to be her dietitian three months prior after a prediabetes diagnosis. We had been meeting weekly.

At our very first session, she told me how twisted the first year of college had been for her. Elena's Mexican immigrant parents were so proud to see her excel in high school and start college yet worried about her rapid weight gain when she came home from semester break. Elena's parents were worried about her health, of course, yet were also worried she would get teased and shut out of opportunities. A trip to the college health center provided Elena and her family with the answer: it was PCOS that was causing the rapid weight gain. That was five years prior to our meeting, and now Elena had to explain to her parents she also had prediabetes.

I learned that Elena's family had a long history of diabetes. Both of her parents lived with it and tried to follow their doctor's direction to eat less carbs and more protein. This led to her family avoiding their staples like tortillas and beans. Elena observed her parents following diet after diet to manage their diabetes, fit in with American foodways, and stuck in their own Diet Trap.

Family dieting led Elena to eat in secret starting in middle school. I noticed carbohydrates were restricted so severely in the home that it was only Elena's self-described binges that were giving her the nutrition she needed for normal puberty. Unfortunately, Elena felt so ashamed of her secret out-of-control eating that eating carbs, fun foods, sweets, or anything not labeled "good" triggered shame and restriction.

Over a three-month period, Elena worked in our sessions to name the harm she experienced from her family's *I-Should-Eat* scripts as well as the oppressive systems that put them there. Xenophobia was particularly problematic for Elena and her family; it made sense to her why her family pushed these food rules. They just wanted her to be safe and belong.

Elena found a rhythm with her CHIPs that calmed her relationship with food and enabled her to feel safe enough to add back foods. This provided a newfound opportunity for exploring Mexican foods that brought her closer to her extended family. Although no longer living, she remembered watching her grandparents prepare family staples in the kitchen and lovingly shoo her away when she tried to help. Elena reconnected with family members who still remembered some of these recipes. She started to be a sort of family food historian, writing down how to prepare these family favorites. I would tear up hearing her joy from these conversations and concrete connections with her ancestors. We knew she was mending her Food Voice with each recipe.

I was reminded again that food is so much more than fuel. It's a part of the collective, grounding us while also uniting us with people who are living on in memories.

Elena explored her cultural foods with excitement for many months then abruptly changed her direction when announcing her intention to start using gentle nutrition. Gentle nutrition is an intuitive eating concept that attempts to weave in anti-diet tools with medical nutrition therapy.[1] Medical nutrition therapy, or MNT for short, comes from nutrition science research and, as a dietitian, represents the pinnacle of my training. If you ever read a food research study headline, you've brushed up against medical nutrition therapy. I always think these headlines make nutrition science sound sexy, yet it really isn't that flashy.

Weaving MNT into finding your Food Voice will be tricky. Nutrition science is not black and white; it is tedious and expensive to study which foods promote health because researchers need to control for genetics, environment, oppressive systems, emotional health, and comorbidities. Because of all these variables, very few nutrition studies show a certain food can *cause* disease; most studies are instead *correlational*. This means a mere relationship is there. It may be easier for you to notice the big difference between correlation and causation using a nonfood example: we wouldn't say a smoker's yellow teeth cause lung cancer; rather the yellow teeth have a relationship with lung cancer because we know smoking is the cause.

All the healthy foods you've learned about in your lifetime are not absolutely healthy but just have a *relationship* with health. Very few of those "unhealthy" or "bad" foods cause direct harm (the exceptions are allergies and intolerances). Even though nutrition research has shown only a relationship with health and food, there's still a place to add it into our lives. Gentle nutrition attempts to add health discussions without triggering the *shoulds* and shame.

Many clients have directed me to teach them gentle nutrition during the last 20 years, and I was not surprised when Elena started the session with that statement.

"I am happy to explore gentle nutrition with you, Elena. First, though, tell me what's been going on and what led you to this next step."

Elena began to describe to me a fun week reconnecting with family during a holiday. They spent hours over leisurely meals laughing and reminiscing. Elena even prepared family recipes that brought joy to her parents. After the holiday was over, Elena went home to her empty apartment with only her leftovers.

"I could not stop thinking about the leftovers. I ate them all at my next CHIP time alone in my apartment," Elena shared. "I *had* to eat them. I wasn't hungry and I felt overfull after. Now I feel like crap. Not just my thoughts but also my body. I noticed I have been more sluggish and can't focus. This isn't right. I can't stop eating, and I can't keep giving myself permission. I need more fruits and vegetables. I need more protein. You need to help me eat healthily now that I have done all this work. It is time for me to pursue health."

I could feel her frustration and overwhelm from across the room. She thought pursuing permission to eat meant she was giving up and losing control.

I shared with Elena that clients often come in after a few months of the work of finding their Food Voice asking for gentle nutrition training. The desire comes in from a thought process I typically find to be premature. This happens for a few reasons including:

- The eating pendulum as described in Chapter 5 and 6 has been pulled away from dieting, spent time in permission, and is now just naturally swinging back toward restriction. This can feel alarming and, at the same time, desperate.
- Practicing permission feels exciting at first then scary. It makes sense that we grasp for concrete scripts disguised as merely gentle nutrition when that fear hits.
- Your scripts have trained you to not trust the healing process but have rather led you to believe that you can only find health outside of your own desires.
- Capitalistically infused healthcare has taught us to prioritize rigid eating plans over healing; physical health over mental health; body size over quality of life. Prioritizing your healing while finding your Food Voice *is* health promoting but the world will suggest otherwise.

If you, like Elena, notice physical discomfort during your CHIPs patterns, you may wonder whether there is anything you can do to lessen or alleviate it. Some of the patterns can be:

- sluggishness
- fatigue
- primal food cravings
- headaches
- restlessness
- dysregulated menstrual cycles
- mood swings
- difficulty sleeping.

Carving out the gentle nutrition nuance intersecting with health comes with curiosity rather than fear. I notice when folks ask to do gentle nutrition work, they are scared. Pursuing gentle nutrition in a spirit of fear has led many of my clients to go back to their scripts. Please be aware that it is a slippery slope. If your brain messages request more balance in your eating or movement, you may be prematurely drawn to gentle nutrition.

After discussing the pros and cons, Elena decided to wait and put gentle nutrition work on pause for a bit longer. A few months later, Elena described going out to breakfast with a friend and eating eggs with her typical oatmeal. She noticed she felt more energized that whole day and experienced less cravings. This experience made her *curious*. Would the same happen if she prepared the eggs at home? When she tried that a few days later and felt the same energy and decreased cravings, she knew she was on to something.

Our next session explored what about that breakfast may have led to improved energy levels and decreased cravings. We considered these options:

- increased protein
- increased fat
- more calories
- more enjoyable
- longer duration
- sweet and salty combo (brown sugar oatmeal and the eggs with salsa).

At this point, Elena and I were just guessing. We wondered out loud whether it was the eggs or components within them. Could she have the same experience with breakfast chorizo? Or avocado toast? Or a quesadilla?

Detaching from the outcome, Elena spent the next week experimenting and taking notes. Her data collection suggested that having protein and fat with her breakfast that also included sweet fiber-rich carbohydrates helped her energy levels and decreased cravings. It didn't seem to matter what the protein and fat choices were as long as they paired carbohydrates with fiber. The rest of our next session Elena asked me questions about how adding fat and protein could impact her PCOS. Could there be a reason? We explored topics such as blood sugar, insulin, and sleep quality.

At this meeting, I heard how compassionate curiosity was directing Elena's nutritional observations about cause and effect. She sounded flexible and okay with any outcome. This felt starkly different from the day she had urgently announced that learning about gentle nutrition would be her next step. That felt like rigid punishment, not caretaking.

Elena noticed foods affecting her differently while finding her Food Voice, and you may as well. I do believe you can include food changes while repairing your relationship with food. Just don't pressure yourself to fix your eating or make it healthier because everyone needs different timelines. I can't predict when you will be ready, if ever, to apply gentle nutrition to your relationship with food. If you push health too urgently, you will more often than not find yourself just following another script. Gentle nutrition can become a prescription, and trying to make it work before you are ready has harmful consequences. You will delay your healing and risk that slippery slope of script thoughts and behaviors.

I told Elena she had completed an interesting science experiment that showed her more data than any other nutrition research. She learned ways to eat that benefited her—specific to her age, ethnicity, cultural background and foods, lived experiences, and chronic health concerns. No other nutrition research can do that.

Curious Nutrition

Adding onto the gentle nutrition concept, I refer to adding new foods through experimentation as *Curious Nutrition*. This is about noticing how food choices impact your past, present, and future self. It also includes detaching from the outcome without urgency. Curious Nutrition uses compassionate curiosity to explore new options. It also has no moral obligation—you are not "good" or "bad" based on food choices. The more experiments you do, the more data you have. You may know eating certain foods may lead to sleepiness or brain fog, and that eating them anyway does not make you a bad person. Sometimes eating a food that may lead to a headache—like a midday slice of birthday cake with a friend—is the kindest choice to allow you to live in the moment, be in *relationship*, feel pleasure, and fuel your body.

Curious Nutrition can very quickly become another *I-Should-Eat* script. So much so that I encourage you to be mindful of its power. When you are drawn to "healthier" eating, you can be walking a tightrope. Fortunately, my clients and I found a loophole to help make this step a bit safer: instead of focusing on what to remove from your eating, focus on what you can add.

Add, not subtract

A quick Google search on food and PCOS will show you 33 million-plus website options on what *not* to eat. People with PCOS get inundated with rigid food rules upon diagnosis (even though no research confirms any diet exists that helps most people with PCOS long-term). No wonder people with PCOS are more likely to live with an eating disorder compared to people without PCOS.[2]

My clients with a dual diagnosis of PCOS and an eating disorder had something in common: they were following their doctor's orders to restrict carbs and sugar and it only led to chaos. Instead of lessening their PCOS symptoms long-term, these scripts just made matters worse. Not only did physical health suffer in the long term, but mental health tanked. On average, it takes someone seven to fourteen years to recover from an eating disorder—a silent, expensive, time-consuming, life-altering relationship killer that breeds shame. These casual food recommendations from healthcare providers impact people's lives and have dire consequences.

I was taught in my dietitian training to treat PCOS with carbohydrate restriction and weight-loss interventions. When I started seeing clients with PCOS regularly, I was already aware of the ineffectiveness of diets and the harm they cause. At the same time, I heard from my clients with PCOS that primal, intense carbohydrate cravings were the norm, yet they were just expected to omit or limit carbs. Even when my clients were able to restrict them as directed by their healthcare provider, the cravings only intensified. I remember Elena describing cravings as if every cell in her body were screaming at her to eat something sweet or starchy or she would die. Eventually, all of my clients with PCOS would eat carbohydrates and feel out of control, ashamed, and sluggish.

I knew there had to be another way. I sought mentors to train me on PCOS medical nutrition therapy that did not push weight loss. Finding someone was tough as this was before any social media and only a baby Google. Thankfully, I connected with Monika Woolsey, a fellow registered dietitian trained in eating disorders willing to look outside of weight loss to treat PCOS. Monika was a wiz at endocrinology and taught me how certain nutrition components are needed because of deficiencies or defects. She also said PCOS carbohydrate cravings were a signal from the body that it lacked certain nutrients; removing carbohydrates would only make things worse.

While the complete PCOS medical nutrition therapy interventions are outside the scope of this book, something in particular changed how I taught Curious Nutrition. Instead of removing carbohydrates, people with PCOS need to add more calories and protein. While some folks need to add more than just those two, thousands of folks found just eating enough and adding more protein weakened or eliminated those primal carbohydrate cravings, regulated cycles, and balanced blood sugar.

I now know cutting out carbs and sugar is like putting the cart before the horse. People with PCOS probably just need more protein and to be sure they are eating enough.

While I appreciate you may not live with PCOS, we can learn from this. Taking away foods probably won't work, isn't necessary, and can cause harm. What if instead we flipped the eating less strategy upside down? While finding your Food Voice, I encourage you to wonder: What can I add rather than subtract?

Before starting your Curious Nutrition experiments

Are you noticing shifting energy patterns, sluggish feelings, headaches, or any other body discomforts? Have you been diagnosed with PCOS, high cholesterol, diabetes, or another chronic health condition? If you have answered yes to any of these, I have written the rest of the chapter for you. I wrote this for you whether you have stumbled upon a certain food impacting your day like Elena or are curious about what you can experiment with.

While some of the following recommendations will be helpful no matter what you are eating right now, none will pale in comparison with eating enough. Getting to the point of eating enough to support your mind and body can take time so I think it is okay to explore some of these experiments, yet just know that the full expression of any food additions won't be felt until you are eating enough.

What is eating enough? That depends, and if you stumble here, working with a non-diet dietitian can help you hunt for your answer. Review Chapter 5's pivot guardrails and add as many as you need.

Over the rest of this chapter, I will describe certain tools to experiment within your day. They are in addition to what you enjoy, have access to, and already include. They are not substitutions. They are not absolute and never required. They are merely suggestions from sitting across from others in a similar place in their Food Voice recovery. I encourage you to skim the headings and only consider the ones that appear helpful and accessible and support your healing. Healing is always the priority, and avoid any suggestion that triggers more script downloads. When you find the triggers, and we all have them, note them. They will be useful while reading the next chapter.

Remind yourself while doing this practice: your Food Voice keeps you out of the Diet Trap, promotes long-term emotional and physical health, and helps set others free.

Does everyone need to do Curious Nutrition experiments?

No.

You never have to explore options to improve health, and you don't have to work on anything else. You have permission to continue to find your Food Voice on your own terms and you don't owe anyone anything when it comes to your personal pursuit of health. Exploring these Curious Nutrition experiments may appear simple yet they are not easy. Weight bias, eating disorders, or other factors disconnecting you from your Food Voice can trigger more trauma when adding in these experiments. While I do explore what to do in these situations in the next chapter, I want you to also appreciate that you are in the driver's seat. You decide whether you'd rather just skip ahead. There is no failure in doing so now or ever. Your worth is just as valid, and you still deserve permission to have an uncomplicated relationship with food.

Setting up your Curious Nutrition experiments

After you have practiced your CHIPs for a few weeks, you may notice some foods help lessen annoying symptoms or energize you differently. When this happens, note it on the "Curious Nutrition experiment" worksheet. This can also be found at FindYourFoodVoiceBook.com or library.johnmurraylearning.com.

Curious Nutrition experiment #_____

Food, movement, or other self-care practice:

What I noticed:

increased energy

more satisfaction with food

better sleep

improved mood

whatever was different

Important data:

time of day

place

alone or with others (and whom)

what I was eating, if anything

other relevant observations

Trigger noted:

observations

While documenting your observations, I invite you to use common scientific language. Researchers use words to convey unbiased observation rather than judgment. If you start writing words like *should*, *I didn't need that*, or *unnecessary* I encourage you to take a step back. Try to find less judgmental language or take a break from this Curious Nutrition experiment. It is okay to take your time or pause experiments indefinitely.

Remember this vital aspect of Curious Nutrition: these experiments add foods, and do not take them away. It's not about eating less of a certain food either; decreasing foods on purpose just makes it another *I-Should-Eat* script.

How many Curious Nutrition experiments can I undertake at a time?

While you may desire a speedy change to symptoms, I find experiments take time and provide the best data when only one is going on. The only exception to this may be the addition of a supplement which I have found to still provide clear data while experimenting with food, movement, or other self-care behaviors.

How long will Curious Nutrition experiments take?

I have been working toward rejecting diet culture since around 2002, and I still run my own Curious Nutrition experiments. I do not undertake them every day, and they no longer need to be written down. You, too, can expect a lifetime of changing food needs. Those of us lucky enough to continue to be alive and have a Food Voice will experience aging. Body changes from the aging process allows for more experiments as our needs change. Change is the only constant, and it is important to remember that when our bodily needs change we are not doing something wrong. We are simply alive.

Each experiment you perform may need a few days' worth of data or more. Try to remain open to flexible data collection while also allowing it to be imperfect.

Example Curious Nutrition observations

Consider the following sample list to stimulate compassionate curiosity and experimentation rather than prescription. Each example observation will include potential positive side effects with adding this to your self-care routine. Be sure to note whether any Curious Nutrition observation activates something within you that feels like a trigger or a fast track to craving a script (this will be useful in the next chapter). If you need food ideas, check out the Food Idea Lists in the appendix.

Adding carbohydrates

I was in the last year of my nutrition undergraduate degree when a family friend asked for my opinion on carbohydrates because she was exploring new ways to promote health.

I told her what I knew at the time:

- Nutrition research taught me needs were met when at least 50 percent of intake included carbohydrates.
- It is the body's preferred source of fuel.
- Carbohydrates provide necessary nutrition including fiber, vitamins, and minerals.

- They allow for better bowel health including the microbiome.
- Athletes and folks who have physically intense jobs will need a much higher percentage of carbohydrates, not a lower one.
- Getting enough helps with focus and mood and promotes better sleep.
- Complex carbohydrates provide long-term energy while simple carbohydrates provide short-term energy; humans need both.

I could see this friend's eyes rolling after just a few of my responses. She said, "I can't believe you are taught this. Have you heard of Atkins?"

Just as I was finishing my nutrition undergraduate degree fats were moving out of the "bad" food category to make room for carbohydrates. The Atkins Diet fast-tracked this change, even though our human nutrition needs hadn't changed. This was especially problematic because every culture around the globe includes a carbohydrate source as a staple. Think tortillas, rice, bread, pasta, naan, and so on—can you think of one culture that does not include a carbohydrate source frequently in its foodways?

From that time period through the early 2010s, I worked with folks with eating disorders who experienced two different types of restriction depending on their age. The over-30 group tended to rely on carbohydrates as the only safe macronutrient because their scripts shamed fat intake. The under-30 crowd feared those carbohydrates as popular diet companies pushed this new selling point and sewed confusion.

These clients restricting carbohydrates ended up being more constipated, sluggish, withdrawn, and distracted than my clients relying on carbohydrates. This happened because the brain prefers carbohydrates. As you challenge your carbohydrate- or sugar-restricting *I-Should-Eat* scripts, look for positive changes to your bowel health, focus, hydration, sleep, and mood.

Adding protein

While the popular opinion on carbohydrates has waned, protein has risen in the ranks as the "in" macronutrient. Protein has important roles, and it is *equally important* to carbohydrates and fats. We all need protein in varying amounts, and some of us will probably need more.

Protein helps our body to build muscles and bones (when there are enough calories along with other nutrients). It also helps make enzymes and hormones. Just like carbohydrates, proteins can be an energy source, yet are not as preferred as carbohydrates.

If you have dieted or restricted for any length of time, your body needs to repair the shredded muscles and bones that helped your body during times of lack. As clients have repaired their complicated food history, I have observed a higher than typical need for protein to repair the inflammation caused by not eating enough. What does this mean? Adding more protein without taking anything away may help your body heal from times of malnutrition.

As I mentioned earlier in the chapter, people with PCOS probably need more protein. I also find folks with insulin resistance and diabetes benefit from a similar recommendation. Adding protein helps insulin do its role in mediating food for cellular energy. You will know whether adding protein is helping your insulin levels when you feel more satisfied at meals, experience less cravings, and more energized throughout the day. You can also test how well your insulin is working to balance blood sugar by taking a HOMA-IR test. This test measures your fasting insulin and fasting blood sugar and puts it through a calculation to determine how much insulin your body needs to lower blood sugar. I find it to be more helpful than just the common A1c typically used.

Adding fat

Where are my Gen Xers and tell me when you learned the myth that fat is bad? I blame the 1990s' Food Guide Pyramid (see Chapter 2) shuffling fats to the pointed top and shapeshifting to a coach wagging his finger while yelling at you to stop eating high-fat foods.

As someone born in the 1970s, I was trained to fear fat and minimize its role in human nutrition. Imagine my surprise when I learned in my nutrition undergraduate studies the vital role fats play in our human existence.

Have you ever found yourself constantly hungry and craving quick-to-digest sweet foods? Like a person on a reality show trying to build a fire using only kindling (and getting kicked off because they lost), the quick-to-digest foods can get things started yet burn out quickly. You can keep adding kindling, yet you will find yourself needing to eat very often, even disrupting your sleep just to eat.

When clients tell me about this type of constant hunger I immediately evaluate for two things:

- Is this person eating enough total calories?
- Is this person including enough fat?

Carbohydrates and proteins fuel our body, yet we also need fat. Fat provides essential building blocks for cell membranes, hormones, and enzymes. It is necessary to absorb vitamins A, D, E, and K. Fat even coats our nerves to help our thoughts and messages move with ease via amazing myelin sheaths. Have you ever followed an *I-Should-Eat* script that left you in a bit of a brain fog? You probably were not eating enough fat, and your poor myelin sheaths were starting to fray.

Fat is more than just fuel. Fat in food provides pleasure and satisfaction. I think of fat sources as the *umph* that is at the heart of any great-tasting meal. That pleasure comes from a complete hunger fullness cycle of hormones; we were literally designed via evolution to complete this pleasure loop many times throughout the day.

While you are benefiting from this satisfying meal, insulin has a chance to move glucose into the cells without spiking. This will be especially helpful if you live with insulin resistance, diabetes, or PCOS. The fat we eat also helps repair diet harm and its corresponding inflammation. Essential fatty acids DHA and EPA fill in the scratches, and smooth over the metaphorical rust caused by too much oxidative stress.

How will you know whether adding fats is helping? Look for more satisfaction after a meal or snack, more mental clarity, improved menstrual cycles, easier mood, and better-quality sleep.

Adding fruits

Elena continued to explore her own Curious Nutrition while finding her Food Voice. She was a high-school teacher and found herself dragging around 2 p.m. every day. After a few months of trial and error, Elena learned that eating enough at breakfast and lunch significantly helped, yet she needed quick energy to get through the last few hours of her workday.

"Are there any foods that can give me energy quickly?" she asked during one session.

I explained: "We get energy from calories and certain foods move through our system faster to help us feel energized. Those foods are made up of easier-to-digest simple carbohydrates or sugar. Think of something you enjoy that tastes sweet—those are options to start with."

Elena and I brainstormed ideas she could access while at school: granola bars, jelly beans, mints, and cookies came out first. These were all foods she could get for free anytime at school and not even worry about packing.

"What about fruit? My school always has a box of leftover canned fruit or whole unpeeled oranges from lunch period. They are sweet, and I like them."

I told how fruit can be a quickly digested snack and an option for this list. It also provides fluid, vitamins, minerals, and fiber. Elena asked, "Does it matter if it is canned or fresh? I think I learned at some point that canned fruit was bad because of the added sugar—is it?"

Canned, frozen, and fresh fruit all provide vitamins and minerals along with other micronutrients. Fruits eaten with the peel usually have a bit more fiber; canned and frozen usually have more vitamins and minerals because they are packed at peak freshness. None is bad, and her body could help direct her to know which helps with energy in the way she was seeking.

"Why do you think my energy levels crash around 2 p.m. every day?" Elena asked. I told her I had some guesses yet wondered out loud whether she had any guesses first. "I assume it's from my PCOS and insulin resistance. I remember you told me insulin levels can spike with PCOS, causing fatigue."

I find painful fatigue to be the number-one PCOS symptom complaint, and it happens often for those with insulin resistance or diabetes, too. Insulin tries to do its job to move energy into cells after eating yet can struggle with these conditions; the body makes more to compensate. This surge eventually overrides the need and leaves more insulin hanging around than needed. Extra insulin tells the body that we need energy stat and can lead to intense cravings and a slump in energy levels. When this happens chronically, the fatigue becomes painful.

"That's my guess too, Elena. I wonder what will happen, if anything, when you experiment with a quick-to-digest snack."

Two weeks later Elena came in with data. She noted that any of the foods we listed during our brainstorm—cookies, canned fruit, oranges, mints, jelly beans, and granola bars—gave her a boost. Some only boosted energy for an hour and a few made her crash worse. She wondered whether adding protein or fat to those particular foods would make a difference. She noted in her journal to try that out if the opportunity presented itself.

The granola bars, canned fruit, and oranges appeared to provide the energy Elena wanted, helping her feel more awake but without a sluggish crash. I pictured all of these foods and wondered out loud what they had in common. I also remembered that Elena had noted including more fiber at breakfast had helped her satisfaction and energy levels.

"Elena, I wonder if your body likes it when you add fiber to what you eat. You have noted this at breakfast and at your afternoon snack. What do you think? Are we on to something?"

Elena agreed. "I am finding that I enjoy the taste of foods that include fiber and they feel energizing after eating them. When I want something that alone makes me feel sluggish, adding foods with fiber seems to help make the food feel okay. I love knowing this about how my body works. It feels powerful!"

Adding fruit may be one way for you, too, to add fiber if you enjoy the taste and it promotes energy levels the way you crave. Be sure to not limit to just fresh fruit; canned and frozen are an accessible option that I encourage you to include in your Curious Nutrition observations.

Besides helping with insulin and blood sugar, adding fruit can also help if you are prone to constipation or hard to pass bowel movements. The type of fiber in fruit softens the stool making it easier to pass. It also helps support your gut microbiome—where bacteria live and need this type of fiber provided by fruits and vegetables. Many people recovering from an eating disorder or the diet industry experience constipation because they have not been eating enough. If this rings true for you, I encourage you to start with fruit before vegetables because of the benefits to your bowel movements.

Adding vegetables

If you had to pick one food to describe healthy eating, you probably would pick vegetables. Luckily for us, one food doesn't make up all of healthy eating and vegetables are not the only way to increase health with food. I find vegetables are the toughest Curious Nutrition category probably because of its often stigmatizing healthy connotation. If you find your scripts activated by the mere thought of adding vegetables—great work. You are doing what you need to do to prioritize healing. I will go through what to do with this type of script activation in the next chapter, yet know one thing: you don't ever have to eat a vegetable again. Seriously.

If you find yourself craving vegetables, or remembering some you used to enjoy, or are curious whether they can impact some of your physical symptoms, let's discuss what adding vegetables can do for you.

Vegetables provide a source of fiber which has the potential to help those with insulin resistance, diabetes, or PCOS. Because fiber functionally slows down digestion, it helps insulin and blood sugar balance out. You will know whether vegetables are helping if you notice more satisfaction at meals, increased energy between meals, and improved sleep at night.

Vegetables provide the body with two different types of fibers: soluble and insoluble. The soluble fibers help soften your stool and make it easier for you to pass it. You will know whether adding vegetables is helping when you notice less constipation or going to the bathroom is just easier.

Insoluble fibers act differently; they add bulk to your stool. This is particularly helpful if you have diarrhea or very loose stools. If you are prone to constipation, adding more insoluble fibers can make your stool even tougher to pass.

For the record, non-starchy and starchy vegetables are all vegetables. Further, you don't have to limit your vegetable intake to fresh; canned and frozen provide for you, too. If you hear your scripts shouting this in the canned food aisle, name its elitist roots. Canned and frozen vegetables are options while also being accessible.

Some folks with a sensitive bowel find how vegetables are prepared makes a difference to their bowel movements. If you have access to them, experiment with cooked versus raw and fresh versus canned or frozen to see whether they make any difference for you.

Some research suggests that adding vegetables provides you with vitamins, minerals, and other micronutrients that help with inflammation and heart health. While you may not notice a physical difference, adding vegetables may help improve your cholesterol levels and inflammation markers on lab tests from your doctor.

Vegetables are not magic, though: there is not enough kale and celery to correct the inflammation and cardiovascular conditions caused by racism and other oppressive systems. If you add vegetables and notice it doesn't help your lab work, please know you are not doing it wrongly. We, as humanity, are doing it wrongly and you deserve more safety.

Adding movement

Your *I-Should-Eat* scripts probably have files of content on ways to move your body. From duration and frequency, to intensity and when to do it, exercise has rigid rules, too. Most people I meet who have dieted have movement rules they've learned in diet books or from family lore or medical providers.

Exercise can quickly become another script and trigger diet trauma. So much so that many people healing their relationship with movement find this takes longer than healing their relationship with food. If this is you, I want to gently let you know you never have to exercise again. You can continue to prioritize healing and choose to not include movement.

What do *you* want to do about movement? If you are interested in starting a *curious movement* observation, I have some places to begin.

Research suggests adding movement can potentially help with:

- improving heart health (lowering blood pressure, lowering cholesterol, and decreasing risk of stroke)
- lowering blood sugar
- improving sleep
- lowering stress
- lessening inflammation
- lowering insulin levels
- improving bone health.

While adding movement has the potential to improve these, keep in mind key factors:

- To see chronic disease improvement with movement, one has to also be eating enough.
- More intense exercise may be fun for some, yet it can worsen inflammation and stress markers for many, especially those with PCOS. If you really love high-intensity exercise, you will need to eat more to counteract the impact of more inflammation.

- More is not better.
- Movement cannot replace the removal of oppressive systems like racism, weight bias, sexism, homophobia, ableism, etc. More exercise will not counteract microaggressions. Do not feel as though you are doing exercise wrongly if movement additions don't improve your chronic disease markers.

My first question for you: Do you crave movement? By "crave" I mean a genuine desire, not another *should*. Maybe you noticed some neighbors laughing while playing pickleball. Maybe you were looking through some old photo albums and saw pictures of you and your siblings running through the sprinkler. Maybe you were inspired by watching that dancing reality show.

If you are craving movement, I encourage you to make a list of types of movement (rather than just exercise) you enjoy or could potentially enjoy. Give yourself permission to ease into this experiment; note how you feel while doing the movement and after. Did you notice any shifts in energy levels? Did it matter if it was earlier or later in the day? Did you notice feeling any shifts in your hunger or fullness levels? How, if at all, did the movement impact your experience in your body (i.e. your body image)? Do you prefer solo or group movement?

I hope you also shake the idea that only certain types of movement count. You don't have to sweat, but it's also okay if you sweat a lot. You don't have to get out of breath either. I hope that, if you choose to explore movement, you find joy in some of the moments. I hope you are okay, too, if there are times when the movement just feels... meh. Movement doesn't *have* to be joyful.

Adding sweet-tasting foods

I have a party trick: name any (and I mean *any*) food and I will name the MANY positive benefits it brings to your existence. This magic typically comes out after I reluctantly let someone know what I do for a living.

Everyone wants to know a dietitian's opinion on what is healthy to eat. Dinner party guests like to do one of two things: "jokingly" hold their belly (large or small) and ask, "Can you help me?" or cover their plate and say "I usually don't eat this. How do you eat so healthily?"

During these predictable scenarios, I try to explain that I am not a "normal" dietitian. I like to help people stop dieting and that all foods, notably even sweet foods, get my thumbs-up. Over the past 20 years the reaction to this has changed:

- ca. 2005: "Huh? Haven't you looked around? We are in an obesity epidemic."
- ca. 2008: "So you promote obesity!?!"
- ca. 2012 (assuming I do this only for thin folks with eating disorders): "Oh, eating disorders are so sad. Isn't it all about control?"
- ca. 2016 (not getting it): "I saw you on that TV show. I mean everyone should feel okay in their body but... not everyone, right?! She needs to eat more healthily, amiright?!"
- ca. 2021 (still not getting it): "Good for you. Diets don't work. What kind of lifestyle changes do you recommend?"
- ca. 2024 (from my hairstylist and hoping not to be an anomaly): "Right on. I am with you on this."

When I say all foods you enjoy can be included, I mean it. I am ready for your pushback and I have a feeling your list includes sweet-tasting foods like doughnuts, soda, pastries, cookies, candy, or any of your sweet cultural foods.

One thing I know to be true: they bring value and adding them to your Curious Nutrition practice may surprise you.

Sweet foods give you functionality: they are often shelf stable and accessible and provide quick energy. I encourage you to keep some handy at work and at home when you have to wait longer than expected and panic hunger hits. I also recommend bringing some with you while traveling. I once was stuck on an airplane tarmac for ten hours with only water and the provided mini pretzel bags. That panic hunger stung for days giving me a killer migraine. Never again.

Sweet foods also bring nutritionally important *warm fuzzies*. Think of these as being like an essential vitamin marked up in the giant supplement aisle. Warm fuzzies connect us with fellow humans in the moment like when celebrating a colleague's birthday by eating cake in the breakroom. They also surge our dopamine and oxytocin hormones; eating a sweet treat that reminds us of home. Warm fuzzies give us pleasure and satisfaction—vital eating experiences signaling eating enough to our endocrine system.

While adding sweet-tasting foods to your Curious Nutrition observations, you may note that you have a tough time stopping their consumption. If you experience this, you did not do anything wrong nor are the sweet-tasting foods bad. This data lets you know you have limited experience with these sweet-tasting foods or limited permission to eat them. If your brain says they are bad, whether you have eaten them often or not, you may find yourself magnetized to their constant consumption. This could be a trigger, and I can help you more with this in the next chapter.

If you experience insulin resistance, PCOS, or diabetes, or are over the age of 40 or so, you may notice feeling different during eating sweet-tasting foods compared to after eating them. This may be especially clear when you eat them without other foods. This can happen as our body ages or we experience changes in insulin functionality. If you notice this, I encourage you to experiment with adding other foods to sweet-tasting foods and/or having them with a meal. Do you notice anything different?

You will know that adding sweet-tasting foods helps when you get a boost of energy, satisfy a craving, or feel a wave of positive emotions. If you get all three, bask in the glory of the nutritional trifecta most only experience with sweet-tasting foods. It's a shame we've been trained to exclude them or feel guilty for keeping them in our life. But we are changing that!

Adding salty-tasting or savory foods

A nutrition professor once said she would never give her children Goldfish crackers. She called them "empty calories" and too high in sodium. That same semester at the same university, I snacked on those crackers while teaching a nutrition undergraduate course. I didn't have kids yet so they were just for me but I already knew I would give them to my kids.

Why? If they are empty calories and are high in sodium?

I eat Goldfish crackers and other salty snacks because they are food. The term *empty calories* grates my nerves because no food exists that only provides calories. Those Goldfish crackers, along with anything else scolded for being *empty*, provide function with that fuel. Whenever we hear the term *empty calories* I hope you can hear the elitism and judgment running through its core.

Salty or savory foods provide necessary electrolytes which can be extra handy on hot days or when you need a shelf-stable snack. I also find salty foods help me manage my chronic migraine; they help treat and prevent my migraine attacks.

Besides electrolytes, salty foods can provide texture to our foods, bringing more satisfaction, pleasure, or relief. Crunchy pretzels when angry hit differently and can be notably soothing. Hot crinkle-cut French fries (with mayo—don't come for me) need no justification for their pleasure. Healthy eating includes pleasure, and adding savory foods may be your fast track to meeting this need.

You will know that adding salty or savory foods helps when you feel that *umph* after an eating experience: you feel more awake or more in tune with expressing yourself in emotional eating.

Adding more fluids

While practicing his CHIPs, Paul (whose dad's diabetes diagnosis got his family dieting) noticed increased thirst. When he brought this information to our next session, he informed me what he had learned over the years about hunger versus thirst. "Is it true that, if I am hungry, I am probably really thirsty? That my *body* confuses hunger and thirst so I should always drink something before eating... just in case?"

Paul knew with one look from me I had opinions on this. Clearly, this popular myth came about because of weight bias; (with sarcasm) *obviously*, as humans we cannot take adequate care of ourselves and mistake a natural, normal craving to eat for a natural, normal craving to drink. These are two basic needs we need to meet every single day, so if there is one thing we all have in common it's experience with hunger and thirst. How did we let society convince us that we are doing it wrongly?

You are the expert of your body. If you feel hunger—however you feel or know it is there—trust it *is* hunger. Hunger does not lie. The same goes for thirst. Paul, like many people, noticed increased thirst while practicing his CHIPs. This happens in part because of increasing self-awareness and just looking around in different moments. Don't feel alone if you start practicing your CHIPs and notice how little fluid you consume—this is very common.

There are no hard-and-fast rules when it comes to increasing fluids. Count any drink whether it has calories or not. You may or may not notice feeling different based on what you choose, and I encourage you to be curious as to why that might happen. As you do more Curious Nutrition, you may find times where a can of regular Coca-Cola hits perfectly whereas another time a cup of ice water is what you need.

You will know that adding fluids has helped when you feel thirst cues lessen, feel more alert during the day, and less sluggish between eating times. Obviously, you will need to use the bathroom more, so you will notice a color change to your urine; it can also lessen constipation and replace fluids lost with diarrhea.

Adding supplements

I used to downplay supplements with my clients. In part this happened because I lived through the decision by the US Food and Drug Administration (FDA) to no longer regulate supplements in the 1990s while getting my nutrition degree. I also downplayed supplements from my ingrained elitism, too. I pushed food first hard for years. As I started to specialize in helping people with PCOS, I quickly changed my tune.

Elena and Matilda complained of intense carb cravings and painful fatigue while living with PCOS. Both were not eating enough and struggling to gain permission to do so. I knew that eating more frequently while adding enough carbs, proteins, and fats would help their energy levels. I knew it would also help their carb cravings lessen.

But that would take time.

Two key supplements helped me get over my belief that food was *always* better: inositol and omega 3. I recommend both to everyone with PCOS right from the beginning because they have the ability to impact cravings and energy levels within days or weeks rather than months to years like food on its own.

If you want to add a supplement or two, I have some recommendations to help you measure if they are worth it. I want to help keep you from getting scammed. Remember, supplements are not regulated in the US, and some manufacturers prey on your vulnerability and desire to feel better.

- Start with one supplement at a time. I encourage you to pick just one and wait two to three months to evaluate if it is helping at all.
- Pick a supplement that includes only one rather than multiple combinations. You want to study how each supplement helps, and

if you pick a combination supplement you will not know which supplement is helping or which is making things worse.

- Try to pick a third-party-tested supplement. In order to know what you are getting, third-party testing verifies the ingredients. This is an expensive certification for a company so not every manufacturer can get it. If the supplement is not third-party tested, be wary and be sure you trust the company.
- Remember, more is not better. Whether it's mega dosing or adding unnecessary ingredients, be sure you are getting the amount recommended. This is where working with a knowledgeable dietitian, naturopath, or coach can help. In particular, I have learned a lot from Kerri Fullerton, a Canadian anti-diet naturopathic doctor.
- Know this takes time. While some supplements—like inositol with PCOS—can impact symptoms quickly, most supplements will take time to improve symptoms. I have observed many people need three to six months to get a picture on whether a supplement is worth taking or not. This could take even longer if you are recovering from not eating enough, dieting, and/or experience the impact of oppressive systems.

When you notice a food doesn't vibe

Rae took the time they needed to mend their Food Voice after diet trauma using their Food Voice Toolkit. After many months of practicing compassion and curiosity, they began Curious Nutrition observations. Rae let me know they found a certain group of foods just made them feel ill. This happened no matter when they ate them and whether by themselves or with other foods.

Rae shared, "After I eat most candy, my tummy hurts and my head aches. I feel lethargic, too. I tried pairing candy with a meal and it still happened. What does this mean? Can I never eat candy again?"

After many Curious Nutrition turns, you too may notice a few foods that don't sit well. By that I mean a food may:

- disturb your GI system (tummy pains, gas, cramping, diarrhea, etc.)
- trigger a headache or migraine
- precede sluggishness.

You may notice a certain food doing this on its own or even when combined with other foods. Does this mean this food is bad? No. Does this mean you are bad for eating it? Absolutely not.

What this means is that you have specific information about how a certain food impacts your physical experience. You have individualized insight that no diet book or health expert could provide. Sometimes this food is expected, and sometimes it is surprising. Even after witnessing folks for 20 years doing nutrition observations, I have not found a way to predict which food provokes these experiences. The only way to get to the information, like Rae did, is through compassionate curiosity without judgment.

Rae and I discussed the new data they discovered about candy. They did notice that their physical symptoms were dose dependent: the more candy they consumed, the worse their body felt.

"What should I do with this information? Rae asked.

I always grimace at a *should*, and Rae laughed when I did with theirs. "I encourage you to use it as information. You may choose to let it inform your food choices, but there may be times when you don't have a choice. No matter what, eating candy is still not bad. It is still neutral, and now you have information about how your body reacts to it before, during, and after consuming it."

After a bit of discussion, Rae named a few new candy principles for them. They included:

Eating it at work will be risky because it could get in the way of getting things done. Eating outside of work will be easier.

While many types of candy were just okay-tasting to Rae, Reese Peanut Butter Cups were their favorite. They decided that, when a craving hit for them, they would proceed to eat them, probably reserving that for nonwork days to be able to rest after.

Rae's nieces loved Halloween and Rae always took them trick or treating. To not have candy at all would impact Rae and their nieces' experience. That was not okay. Rae decided to pick the candy they loved—mostly Reese Peanut Butter Cups—and savor the before and during experiences. Even with an upset stomach, that candy helped them connect in that moment.

Dear Struggling for Life,

We wish this world understood and took care of people with different bodies, abilities, and chronic conditions. We also wish you weren't taught to blame your eating when these differences showed up. There was a reason you couldn't control what you ate: it is not meant to be controlled. Like breathing every day, you have successfully taken care of your body by eating. Even when your health is complicated, you still deserve to feel at home in your body and have a pleasurable safe connection with food. Practice that permission and, when ready, curiously experiment with different choices. Remember, there is no right or wrong. There is no perfection or overindulgence. Collect how your body responds to choices—Does your energy shift? Do cravings lessen? Does cholesterol change? Your data will be your own, so perfect for you. No one can take that away.

Love,
Food

Dear Food letter activity

Write a letter to Food describing what you are curious to add to your eating and movement, if anything. How will this practice affirm your Food Voice instead of chip away at it?

References

1 Tribole, E., & Resch, E. (2020). *Intuitive Eating: A Revolutionary Program That Works*. St Martin's Essentials.
2 Lee, I., Cooney, L. G., Saini, S., Sammel, M. D., Allison, K. C., & Dokras, A. (2018). Increased odds of disordered eating in polycystic ovary syndrome: a systematic review and meta-analysis. *Eating and Weight Disorders—Studies on Anorexia, Bulimia and Obesity* 24(5), 787–97. https://doi.org/10.1007/s40519-018-0533-y.

8

Mend

Dear Food,

Since I was a little girl, everyone in my life told me not to eat too much of you, not at the wrong time, not the "unhealthy" versions of you, which according to my mom was almost everything, and definitely don't ask for seconds. I was told that my family didn't like fat people. I was asked if that version of you fit into my diet. I was asked if I was TRYING to gain weight. I don't have any memory at all of having peace with you.

When I was 35, I was diagnosed with PCOS. The doctor told me to cut out a lot of versions of you and put me on medication that made me sick. I found a great diet and lost a lot of weight, but I was starving. I felt hungry all the time. I was craving you but denying you. Then the dam broke and all I did was eat you but in secret. Then you became another problem. An eating disorder.

At 48 I was diagnosed with OCD. I suffered so long before I knew. Then I started to heal.

I gave up the diets and gained some weight. It hurt. I was scared. But I wasn't hungry.

Food, now I eat way too much of you. And I eat foods that don't make my body feel good. When I think of eating something healthy, the alarm bell goes off. It says... hungry! restriction! and don't tell me what to do!

I would like a middle ground with you, Food. To feel some peace and to help my body feel great.

Can we make a compromise?

And how?

Thanks,
Struggling for Too Long

Please note that this chapter names specific traumas that may be unsettling to some. Please take care of yourself as you decide how to move through it.

The five basic human needs

Three days after giving birth, I walked around my hospital room topless and in tears. My nipples were bleeding as I continued to unsuccessfully try breastfeeding my newborn. Someone walked into my hospital room, yet I couldn't see who it was because I had forgotten to pack my glasses and hadn't bothered putting my contacts in. I couldn't care less anyway because I was sobbing uncontrollably.

I cried because I was trying to breastfeed my newborn and couldn't. I was in physical pain because no one prepared me for the possible discomfort of breastfeeding. Why didn't I just offer a bottle? I am a bit weary of admitting this now: as a dietitian, I felt I *had* to breastfeed. (I did indeed formula-feed my second child and it was a much easier newborn period for me. Lesson learned.)

I remember being very emotional, and I blamed that on hormone shifts. As the person entering my hospital room got closer, I squinted to read their name tag. When she was close enough for me to shake her hand, I saw her name was Barb and she was a lactation consultant.

"Just the person I need!" I declared. I told her about my trouble feeding and got so emotional describing the overwhelm and pain.

She kindly offered advice to help with placement and to prevent the pain. As her advice started to work and my daughter was eating, I got to chatting with Barb.

Barb and I chatted about hospital life, and the small talk felt comforting. She asked me how I felt with my new little bundle. "Overwhelmed. Weepy. Anxious. I hate this negative talk too because it was not easy for me to get pregnant, and I don't know if I ever will again."

Barb gently observed that I was putting a lot of pressure on myself. She asked, "What plans do you have to take care of yourself at home?"

I told her how little sleep I was getting at the hospital. I was hopeful I would get more at home without the beeps and other hospital noises.

Flash-forward to a month later and I still didn't get much sleep. My daughter loved to be held and when we put her down she would cry.

Flash-forward to *six* months later and she still wasn't sleeping through the night. I was a mess. This time of my life I was not pleasant to be around. I was grateful to be this baby's mom *and* exhausted. I was cranky, short-tempered, and getting sick often.

I slept in two-hour chunks while trying to work during the day. If you were a client of mine at the time, you probably remember how obsessively I spoke about sleep. I couldn't shut up about it. If you had children, I analyzed how you were able to get your babies to sleep through the night. If you didn't have a child, I wanted to know what it was like to sleep all night and wake up without an alarm. I wanted your sleep details. I had the same conversations with people in the grocery checkout line, the pediatrician's office, and in the playground.

Was I addicted to sleep? Did I have a pathological relationship with sleep? Did I have a problem because I could not stop thinking about and craving sleep? Of course not. I was textbook sleep deprived. And it wasn't going to take just one nap to help me recover. I needed a good year of regular consistent sleep to feel like myself again.

Over time, I thought less about sleep yet still did get an adrenaline rush whenever moms would talk about sleep. I had opinions and loved sharing them. In 2016, I started the *Find Your Food Voice* podcast (called *Love Food* back then), and in the first 20 episodes or so I talked a LOT about sleep even though my first child had been sleeping well through the night for years.

You probably know we need sleep to survive. It is one of the five basic needs we all have as humans to stay alive. The five basic human needs are:

1 sleep
2 hydration
3 oxygen
4 shelter
5 food.

Our five basic needs have three commonalities including:

- predictable intense cravings—thoughts will flood the brain with these cravings when there is a sufficient lack of the basic need
- the brain fixates on this basic need until the need is met, and usually for a while after

- physical symptoms of lethargy, irritability, and emotional outbursts while lacking consistent access to the basic need.[1]

Have you ever visited the desert? I used to have family in Phoenix, Arizona, and loved visiting the desert every March. It wasn't too hot yet and the nights were cool. Each year, I would land at that airport and drive to my family's home already thirsty. It took just minutes for my body to register that I had left my normal humid climate for this desert air.

By the time I completed the hour's drive from the airport to the place I was staying, I had a headache and was cranky. I immediately craved water and could not get enough. The whole trip had me worried that, if I didn't have a water bottle with me, I would regret it. I fixated on water.

Was I obsessed with water? Was I addicted to water? Did I experience a pathological connection to hydration?

Of course not. I was dehydrated. My body told me it needed to be consistently provided with hydration and had predictable signs and symptoms when it was in danger of not getting enough fluid.

Like sleep, hydration is another basic need for every human. When we do not get enough sleep, or any other basic human need, our bodies will respond in predictable ways.

I appreciate you feel shame and blame when food thoughts consume you. People on social media like to call it *food noise* and see it as proof of an individual lacking something. There are plenty of books and podcasts about overcoming these burdens through corrective mindset, brain power, and toxic positivity. Some use GLP-1s—diabetes medications used at higher doses to promote weight loss in people without diabetes—to make it go away. I see healthcare providers teaching people that, if they are obsessed with food, that means they are addicted to it. Or, it means they have a pathological relationship with food.

Food is one of the five basic needs. When you don't get enough or are even *threatened* to not get enough, you will have a predictable response.

- You will crave food. The cravings will be intense and your brain will focus on that craving for food until you eat.
- Your brain will think about food even after eating it. It will need time to consistently receive this food and enough of it before the craving subsides.

- You will be cranky, irritable, and lethargic while craving food. Even the mere possibility of not getting enough food can trigger these mood shifts.

When you experience these predictable responses, you are not doing anything wrong. On the contrary, these responses are so predictable that we know they come from evolution. You literally are being a successful human. Your body and mind are wired to protect you from lacking access to food. It is dangerous to go without food just like it is dangerous not to breathe or have shelter.

That's why when food is withheld for any reason, you experience trauma.

Why is dieting traumatic?

If we heard a story about someone almost drowning, we would be quick to name that experience as traumatic. We all can appreciate how vital air is, and to have that suddenly taken away—even if we have never experienced it—can easily be categorized as catastrophic.

We could say the same about having to live without shelter or without potable drinking water. As I type these words, I appreciate there are many people experiencing this right now and my soul aches thinking about it.

Does your soul ache thinking about food being withheld because of a self-imposed diet? I can appreciate this may not feel as oppressive as lacking oxygen or a safe place to live. But just because something is not the most traumatic, does it mean it isn't tragic at all?

I have some guesses as to why dieting is not labeled as a trauma. For one, many people diet so we have normalized dieting's existence. So many diets exist in the public consciousness that the pain they cause can be quickly minimized and brushed aside. Because hunger is flippantly regarded as not that big of a deal, we get the instruction that it is necessary and that lack of satisfaction is our punishment. We earned this pain. We deserve this pain.

Nutrition science has been oversimplified as just a matter of will and simple math calculations. I remember seeing a diet company ad that read: "It's not rocket science, stupid." We are conditioned to believe how we choose to eat is just functional and a matter of knowledge. The diet industry has taught us that our intellectual proof is supposed to be in our body size. We learn that, if we are smart enough, we should be slimmer by now, dammit, and we would eat the amount that makes our bodies acceptable. What if you will never be white, thin, straight, cisgender, and/or able-bodied? Certain bodies are expected to live constantly experiencing this trauma and stuck in the Diet Trap.

When each *I-Should-Eat* script predictably ends, we are told we didn't try hard enough and we are broken. If we argue in any way, we are told we are mentally ill as well as in physical danger if we don't oblige. It's like being told drowning is the only way to breathe the right way and to stop would be a marker of an unfit mind and body.

Forcing us to abstain from food becomes even more traumatic due to the *food is medicine* and *food is fuel* mantras. If everyone just ate the correct way, I suppose we would always look the same and never die.

What is the correct way? Most media outlets and dietitians preach the white version of the Mediterranean diet full of lean proteins, whole grains, fruits, and vegetables. Cultural and regional foods from Black, Indigenous, and people of color's foodways are now considered wrong in nutrition science circles. People are encouraged to remove them. Food as pleasure, connection, sustainability, and accessibility are quickly disregarded to funnel all of us into eating one *I-Should-Eat* script.

If we cut through all of the fluff, *diet* trauma says: "If your body is not thin, not able, not straight, not white, then you deserve to only eat certain foods at certain times. Does this hurt? Too bad. Are you distracted from things that matter? Too bad. Do you miss certain foods? If you try enough you can earn them back… but not too much. Are you feeling isolated? You must do what it takes to have that body that proves health."

Relying on systemic weight bias rooted in racism, certain bodies are regarded as eating wrongly just by appearances. In the end, we know eating less will never lead to that body, especially the further you are from that white, thin, cisgender, able body. This heartache and torture will be lifelong unless we name the trauma happening right now.

Your body has predictably responded to not getting enough food. These responses have already coded dieting as a trauma. Your body has evolved just like everyone else to require food as a basic daily human need. That need does not change based on what you ate yesterday or whether your clothing size went up. Your basic human needs are constant. Your scripts have led you to believe you are less human and require less. *That is the lie.*

That lie is where the diet trauma begins. Uncovering the falsehood and naming its origins in systemic oppression is the start, yet does not repair the work from the trauma. Even more, the trauma is ongoing since we live in a world where an unchecked diet industry calls the shots. The swirling oppressive systems parading as healthy eating continue to shove you into a cold and turbulent sea. Your scripts expect you to have a smile on your face while gasping to stay alive, thanking the diet industry for holding you underwater every chance it gets.

The difference between famine and choosing to diet

When I first explained the concept of diet trauma to Rae (who had started experiencing this trauma at five years old via their pediatrician), they looked puzzled.

"But I chose not to eat as much. Surely my body reacts differently to a diet compared to a famine?"

While experiencing food insecurity from poverty or war has more complex layers to its trauma, Rae's body did not know why Rae wasn't getting enough to eat. Malnutrition is malnutrition. The body will respond in the same predictable way with increased cravings, distractedness, irritability, and trouble stopping once it gets the food it craves.

After I explained this to Rae, their face went from puzzled to squinting to a softer gaze. Rae stared straight ahead yet I knew their brain was processing their food experiences. They started to nod their head and look around. They took a deep breath in. Rae's soft gaze slowly looked down and met their hands. I knew without seeing them that tears were forming.

There are moments in therapy sessions when you feel a shift happening across the room. As a witness to those moments, I feel the privilege to be sitting across from you holding the space while you are sitting on my green couch (even if this is just figurative while reading this book). I appreciate the religious undertones to the word *sacred*, yet it's the only word I can think of in these moments; they feel sacred. Rae connecting with the concept of diet trauma and identifying it as their experience was one of these sacred shifting moments.

Rae was viewing their relationship with food through a new lens that flooded it with compassion. Rae cried for a few minutes, and when they looked up, their eyes met mine. "That's exactly it. Diets have traumatized me all these years. They still do."

I said, "It looked like I witnessed a shift a moment ago. Did I?"

"Yes. I can't believe all that I have been through. I am so much stronger than the world has told me I am. And now that I see how it has traumatized me, I won't let it tell me anything different. Even though I am crying, I feel powerful."

I hope you, too, feel powerful connecting with the concept of diet trauma. Holding trauma and power together feels clunky, doesn't it? It feels like the two should be diametrically opposed, yet naming your trauma lays down another piece of your personal blame. It names the offender, and it was never you. It names what needs to change, though you can't undertake that change alone. It's not your individual burden. Now that you know about your personal diet trauma, you can help others experiencing the same. And this knowledge is how we will change it for everyone.

That's our power.

How do you know if you've experienced diet trauma?

Paul, who no longer referred to himself as a food addict, knew something was up after a weekend full of green juicing and a trendy online diet forum deep dive. He emailed me Sunday night to see whether he could come in during his Monday lunch hour. This email was a surprise because we had not met in a few months; we had moved our sessions to just quarterly check-ins.

"Only if you bring your lunch, too," I directed.

Paul looked defeated walking into my office with his takeout container with the easy-to-spot diet-coded baked chicken and veggies. "Something's wrong," he admitted while sitting down, "but I am not sure what's happening."

Paul explained that he had been feeling at ease with food the last few months until last week. His coworker was enjoying a green smoothie from a new place near his office, and it looked interesting.

"I hadn't had anything like that in a long time, and it looked like it would taste good. I tried a sip and it did. Later on that day I went down to get the same smoothie for a snack and noticed how great it tasted and how energized I felt afterward."

Paul told me how, a few hours later while waiting for a client meeting to start, he found himself eyeing a plate of doughnuts. He enjoyed some sweets yet doughnuts were not his favorite, especially ones that had been sitting out for hours and were already stale. A coworker saw him looking at them so offered him one. Paul took it and ate it. "I remember feeling satisfied yet also not. I was physically full—really full—yet wanted more."

Instead of focusing on the important work meeting, Paul found himself obsessing over how to get more of the doughnuts without anyone noticing. "I remember being worried that I wouldn't get anymore. Like that one was it." When his coworker left the room, he quickly ate another then grabbed two more and wrapped them in napkins for later.

"They weren't even good doughnuts! But for some reason my mind fixated on them as if they were the last food available on earth."

Paul's brain did think they were the last food on earth because that green smoothie had activated his past diet trauma. In that moment, his brain sounded an alarm letting the rest of his body know that another famine was on its way. Prepare for another diet assault.

"I feel so stupid," Paul said, his voice cracking a bit. "I don't know what is wrong with me but I just ruined all my work this past year with food."

"You didn't ruin anything, Paul," I said. "Your body remembers your past diets and it is trying to protect you. You are not failing; you are showing your body's evolution. Something about that green smoothie pushed a button letting your brain know another diet is coming. This sent messages to your brain to fixate on the foods that will soon be on the forbidden list. I am assuming your past with this trendy diet did not include doughnuts?"

Your body remembers your complicated history with food even if you are years out of relying on *I-Should-Eat* scripts. Eating disorder therapists in recovery and fat activists securely rejecting diets will tell you diet trauma activation can happen no matter how secure you feel around food. How will you know if you are rubbing up against your diet trauma?

Like Paul, you may notice sudden fixated thoughts or feelings about a certain food. You may also notice cravings for certain behaviors like restriction, bingeing, overexercising, or other behaviors you may have used. Matilda, tortured by PCOS diets for years, felt the craving to binge just thinking about adding more vegetables to her Curious Nutrition observations. You, too, may notice the mere thought of eating certain foods connected to your dieting days will trigger your thoughts to be rigid, preoccupied, or fearful.

Food is a basic human need, and every cell in your body remembers how you survived going without enough food. Your body will do whatever it takes to keep you alive even if the threat doesn't feel real to you. Remember, this is a strength not a weakness. This is your mind, body, and soul on your side rooting for you to continue to reject your *I-Should-Eat* scripts.

What to do with activated diet trauma

When you notice activated diet trauma, I encourage you to try to slow down and work through these steps. Go to FindYourFoodVoiceBook.com or library.johnmurraylearning.com for the Diet Trauma worksheet I have created for you.

1 Name it

Feminist theorists teach us to name our experiences and what harms us. By naming the diet trauma infused with your complicated history with food, you place the blame where it needs to be. Remember, this isn't your burden to carry alone, rather an identifiable problem within society. Moving forward, naming your diet trauma out loud will keep you from turning to shame and help you hold on to more power.

2 Accept what is

You may want to resist the idea that "just a diet" traumatized you. Is a diet really harmful, especially when we know how quick healthcare providers, work colleagues, and family members are to direct us in how we should eat? People are fast to cross our personal boundaries and recommend we eat differently. Yes, this is absolutely normal, and that is why diet pushers traumatize us. Our default settings were manipulated to believe we cannot be trusted around food and that it must be regulated in order for us to be acceptable. If you live with multiple marginalized identities, this will be even more rigidly protected as a truth. Recognize that eating enough food is your basic human right. Anyone or anything that blocks that right has caused harm.

3 Ask yourself a question

When a Curious Nutrition observation activates a diet trauma, ask yourself: What is this fear waking up? Paul enjoyed eating a food with a healthy connotation but it activated his diet trauma history. His brain remembered each previous restrictive period started with more vegetables. Drinking the green juice was the only reminder his body needed to sound the alarm and seek enough food while he could.

I mentioned this to Paul at that session: "I wonder what your fear is waking up." After just a few moments, he said, "Every diet started with eating 'very healthily', which for me meant that vegetables were the only thing I would eat in front of others. For a few days I would eat only vegetables and a few other diety foods at home yet eventually I would binge. I see now the binges are how my body got enough when dieting. Just eating that green smoothie my body went into protection mode. It was scared I was doing it again. My body was scared it wouldn't get enough."

I praised Paul for connecting these dots: "This is hard work, Paul. There are many variables and pressures keeping you from connecting with your truth. Your body remembers your past diet trauma and just wants you to be safe. Cuing the binge craving was an act of safety."

"Does that mean I will never eat a vegetable again? Or anything labeled healthy?" Paul wondered.

4 Give permission

While many people can find ways to mend past diet trauma and eat activating foods, I encourage you to have permission not to eat them again. You have a choice here. It is okay and healthy to prioritize healing over eating certain foods or exercising a certain way. Eating enough food is a basic human need whereas eating a certain amount of "healthy foods" or exercising a certain way are not basic needs. Your body may physically benefit from adding certain behaviors, yet you are not a test tube or a robot. You are first and foremost a human being navigating this complex world. Practice giving yourself unconditional permission to not add certain foods or exercise behaviors and you will give yourself space to heal. Does this mean you will never try again? No. But it does leave that as an option.

While most people will, over *time*, find a way to incorporate any food or exercise behavior back into their lives, I have worked with a number of people who found specific foods or behaviors that could not be incorporated into their life without activating diet trauma responses. For them, they have moved past the pressure to include these changes in favor of mental health and healing. I hope you, too, can do this. You deserve to feel as safe as possible within your body, especially while meeting your basic human needs. This is your right, and no vegetable deserves to trump that right.

5 Try to be patient

Matilda felt her diet trauma activated just by thinking about adding certain foods. If you have followed *I-Should-Eat* scripts for years, I expect this to happen to you as well. The mere thought of less food is enough for the human brain to fixate on your basic need. After the first time her diet trauma was triggered, Matilda backed off and gave herself permission to wait. She wasn't happy with waiting, rather felt inpatient. I let her know that mending the diet trauma harm takes longer than we think it will, and it is worth it to take your time.

A few months later, she was invited to a meeting that provided lunch. She found out the night before the lunch was a salad bar, a staple during her dieting days.

"I felt my fear when I saw the lunch menu, and I knew it was waking up my past scripts," Matilda told me. As she noticed the fearful panic, she put her hand on heart and felt her heart beating. This grounded her. She told herself she was safe, and she would give herself enough to eat. Just in case the salad didn't provide enough options, Matilda decided to bring some crackers and trail mix along with something sweet. As she packed these items the night before, she felt the anxiety start to fade. Can you see how Matilda used the same tools you've learned—getting grounded, connecting with your Food Voice, and planning for permission to eat enough—to help repair her diet trauma? You can do this, too.

Be patient while you are mending. You may need repeated exposures to what is activating your diet trauma in order for your brain and body to feel okay moving forward. You also may need to collect more data to understand what you need in order to not be fearful. Like Matilda, you may need grounded reassurance that you will have access to enough food. This may mean packing extra snacks or eating something before. Figuring out what you need takes time, but I promise it is worth the time spent.

Other common diet trauma examples

My clients and I find the topic of diet trauma can be hard to pinpoint until we are right in front of it. Still confused about the concept of diet trauma? Wonder what actually can be done about it? Consider these common examples I have seen in my practice and the ways folks have seen them through. This may or may not exactly ring true for you or miss the mark altogether. That's okay. I hope they help you clarify your experience and help you mend wherever you are in the moment.

Eating one specific food previously labeled as safe

While rigidly following a previous script, many past clients had "safe" foods. These were foods eaten by themselves every day, sometimes many times a day, because of following certain rules. Traci, the teen client who struggled to recover from her eating disorder and the anger that came with it, had a specific safe food. While entrenched in her eating disorder, she ate at least two pears every day and tried to convince me they were plenty for a meal or snack. While they undoubtedly were not, pears were giving her some nutrition, so we kept them and added yogurt, nut butters, and crackers to her early meal planning. Eventually, whole meals and snacks were built on the backs of these pears. I knew she was starting to heal her brain when she told me how tired she was eating these dang pears. "Can I have something else? I am so bored of them!"

Traci added new things to her eating and eventually didn't need a meal plan anymore rather just relied on her CHIPs. A few years later, no longer needing CHIPs, she came into my office looking defeated. She explained that, while hanging out at her friend's house, she had had a pear for a snack.

"Immediately, I knew something was wrong. I started to worry about the pizza we had just ordered. I decided I would only eat one piece ... then decided I would take off all the toppings ... then couldn't even eat it when it arrived. My friend was so confused. I lied and said I didn't feel well and drove home. What the hell is wrong with me?!"

Pears were Traci's diet trauma activator. Holding, tasting, and smelling that pear was enough to reactivate her *I-Should-Eat* script and send her back into its rigid controlling rules.

We discussed ways to try the pear again in case she wanted to incorporate it. She could cut up a few pieces as a part of a bigger meal or she could bring a few pears to session for us to eat together. After discussing what to do about this over many sessions, Traci decided she didn't want to ever try a pear again. "My recovery is too important to risk another slip."

It has been over a decade since I worked with Traci. I have no idea whether she ever ate a pear again, but whatever she chose next I am rooting for her. In the same way, I am rooting for you whether you decide to continue avoiding certain food or to find a workaround. How you repair is up to you and only you.

Joining an exercise program

There's something about joining a running training program or doing a bootcamp that lights up the diet trauma alarms. Why? I am guessing it's the coach-like loud enthusiasm, the motivating high fives, and the disguised shame. Recovering from diet trauma related to movement can be the toughest to recover from, and I hope you know that if you experience this you are not alone. Does this mean you will never move your body again? For most people they will recover their relationship with movement through redefining it. If you find yourself triggered like Traci was with her pear after starting a new exercise option, I encourage you to give yourself permission to explore other options. For many people, movement needs to include three Ps to prevent a trauma activation: people, places, and play.

- **People:** Solo exercise can be especially triggering through its isolation. I find it to be a funnel to scripts. A gentle rule may be for movement to include other people. This could be a hiking club, a rumba class, or pickup soccer.
- **Places:** Gyms have diet goals all over them. Just walking into them I can feel the pressure to pursue weight loss and that is often reinforced by words overheard and messages splashed across posters. Many clients over the years have found safety by simply not joining a gym. Others have opened fat-positive gyms prioritizing safety.
- **Play:** No pain no gain—no thanks! Many clients activated by exercise have opted to include play as a requirement in movement. Some need full-on laughter when hula hooping whereas others stick to games like softball, basketball, or another team sport with friends. Bonus points when this laughter turns into community and meals afterward.

Panic hunger hits

Hunger in its most intense forms can be quite uncomfortable for most of us. We feel light-headed, nauseous, and irritable along with wanting to consume everything around us. Extreme hunger hurts because our body wants us to eat to meet one of those basic needs. While CHIPs and consistent access to food help us prevent panic hunger, we can't always avoid it.

You, too, may find yourself unexpectedly stuck on airport tarmac like me after a short flight with only mini bags of pretzels for hours. You, too, could forget your wallet and money when showing up for jury duty and be stuck waiting for hours without access to food.

Whatever the reason, waiting too long to eat and cuing that primal panic hunger pushes that diet trauma button for many people. If it does for you, you may find yourself bingeing or, the flip side, restricting more. Something to note, too: I see panic hunger activating diet trauma responses in folks with a past history of food insecurity from poverty or neglect as well as from dieting.

If intense hunger triggers a diet trauma response in you, try to notice it and connect the dots. While that is not always possible in the moment, it can be a few hours or days later, especially with repetition. I encourage you to remind yourself that panic hunger is a normal protective part of your evolution and that how you are responding is, too.

Consider adding shelf-stable food to your pantry and your car. Stash some easy-to-carry food in your work bag or office drawer. You may not need them very often, yet seeing them there will reassure you that you have consistent access to them.

Do you still experience food insecurity from poverty or neglect? I want to fix that. Those of us reading this book with access are working to end food insecurity; this isn't your burden to fix. Please be kind to yourself when your body protects you and feels out of control around food. You are not doing anything wrong; rather our world is.

Eating to fullness or feeling out of control while eating

Fullness sensations are meant to be reassuring, pleasurable, and satisfying. Unfortunately, we live with the diet industry's influence telling us lies about not deserving these perks. Rae taught me how intertwined fullness and shame felt to them. As we worked in sessions to neutralize that shame, they found that feeling full cued diet trauma.

"As soon as I feel really full—like 8 or 9 out of 10 on the hunger fullness scale—I feel like a pig and as though I have no self-control. A part of me knows this is wrong, yet a part still believes this."

If you, too, notice a diet trauma response when very full, I hope you can consider what that part believing these false beliefs needs. It may need reassurance your worth has nothing to do with how much you eat or weigh. It may need reassurance that you no longer have to perform to access joy. Like those with activated diet trauma from panic hunger, that part may need a visual reminder you will continue to have access to enough food.

Eating past fullness or feeling out of control with food is to be expected while finding your Food Voice. With repetition, the experience will teach your brain and body that you do not have to be as guarded around food. Your brain and body will start to appreciate it isn't figuratively drowning anymore and you can breathe normally. Some of the toughest moments, though, can be when an out-of-control eating experience occurs out of the blue. If it has been a while, and the amount of food and the intensity of the feelings may be more than ever before. Please know that is the textbook way I notice most people recovering their Food Voice. To help you move forward, I encourage you to notice it happening as soon as you can then name it. Deliver an abundance of compassion and try to be patient. You have not ruined anything; rather you have been given a new set of data.

Even more, out-of-control eating experiences are typical for most humans every once in a while. This means that even if someone has never dieted or experienced diet trauma, one could still binge or feel out of control while eating. The difference is they do not connect it with shame because no one has taught them to do that. While that may feel impossible to imagine, you can still access the option to reject the shame. Remember, the shame isn't yours but rather belongs to the oppressive systems trying to control you.

Thinking about starting a new *I-Should-Eat* script

You read this correctly: just thinking about eating less is enough to activate a diet trauma response within you. I have lost count of the number of people who've told me they noticed more binge eating or another behavior tied to their script history after just thinking about a diet. These dreamlike diet fantasies begin when cued by something outside of a person's control:

- Scheduling a big event like a wedding or class reunion where you will see people you haven't seen in a while.
- Experiencing a microaggression connected to your script development history.
- Reading a work announcement for an office "Wellness Challenge" or weight-loss competition.
- Living through January, aka International Dieting Month.

When you connect the dots that your thoughts are circling around the possibility of eating less, congratulate yourself for the awareness. Give yourself compassion that the world neglected to provide. Reject the notion that there is something wrong with you unless you show up smaller. When that rejection feels inaccessible, give yourself even more compassion and know I am rooting for you. You haven't ruined anything but are rather finding ways to survive. That, my dear Voice Finder, is your superpower.

Dear Struggling for Too Long,

We see the constant emotional roller coaster the diet industry and eating disorder have caused you. You have been traumatized. With each eating opportunity that ends up with a belly ache, please know this is you and your mind attempting to heal. It is waking up a fear. You deserve peace and safety every time you eat. You deserve to know you can always have enough food. For now, it may feel too much or never ending. Practice compassion, especially in the moments when food feels out of control. That is where the wound lives, and it needs attention when you can consider its message. There's no way to know how long this recovery will take, yet know you deserve every second it takes.

Love,

Food

Dear Food letter activity

Write a letter to Food describing your diet trauma history. Include only the bits you find helpful to record. Let Food know you see now how it was neither you nor Food doing it wrongly. Describe what you need to patch up the hurt this diet trauma caused. What can you use to patch it up?

Reference

1   Kater, K. J. (2005). *Healthy Body Image: Teaching kids to eat and love their bodies too!: promoting healthy body image, eating, fitness, nutrition and weight: a comprehensive resource manual and lesson guide with scripted-lessons and activities for grades four, five or six.* Eating Disorders Awareness and Prevention, Inc.

9

Nest

Dear Food

I've had a long uphill battle with you over the last number of years. I blamed you for everything wrong with my body, and my life. I struggle each and every day as a fat person living in today's world. It's so much easier to blame food and the desire for food than go against the crowd and say that diets and culture are the problems, even though that's what I really believe. I feel so alone in the fight to raise awareness of fat phobia, anti-fat bias, and the relationship between fat bodies and eating disorders. In fact, most people I decided to disclose my eating disorder to had a preconceived idea of what I was about to tell them.

- I'm fat, so I must binge eat.
- I'm fat, so I can't possibly exercise.
- I'm fat, so I must only eat high-fat/carb/calorie/whatever label foods.
- They somehow try to relate to me by saying that they can't control their desire to eat either.

What is more astonishing is their reaction when I tell them that I starved myself for years, that I spent more hours a day exercising and/or thinking about exercise than I did doing anything else, that I destroyed my GI system by purging and abusing medications that were never meant to be used to aid in losing weight. They don't understand how much effort it took to get where I'm at now, much healthier and more in tune with my body. They also don't understand that I have to plan meals for the week or I won't eat; or that going to the grocery store sometimes causes panic attacks. They get offended when I choose not to eat around them because of their negative food and weight comments that shame me into silence and avoidance. Recovering from years of self-hatred and self-abuse means that I have to put in extra effort to make sure I don't go backwards. No matter how much I try to explain, most don't understand it.

All this to say, food, is that I'm tired. I'm tired of fighting a battle very few people truly understand. I'm tired of keeping silent when people demonize and weaponize food. I'm tired of smiling when people make comments about food just to avoid a conversation I know will cause me distress. I just want the world to understand that people in fat bodies are humans, too. We deserve to be treated with respect. Our experiences are valid.

Sincerely,
One exhausted human
KJH

In March 2020, I was lucky enough to be able to work from home while living through the COVID-19 pandemic. As I reluctantly homeschooled my kids and shared office space with my then partner, my front porch became my favorite place. That year in particular was not as rainy so I was able to spend a lot of time there just sitting in the sun. Nature grounded me and helped my extroverted self connect with my neighbors walking by.

During this period, I noticed bluebirds nesting in my front yard. I had four nest boxes spread out within eyesight. As those long days ticked by, I monitored the male bluebirds preparing their nest with each swoop-in with material. They would disappear for a moment inside the box and reemerge moments later to get more.

I still get a bit of a dopamine rush when I see a bluebird: I have learned they are not ones to mingle and we have to look for them. Their feathers remind me of my favorite blue highlighter in high school because it, too, was so bright you couldn't miss it once you started noticing.

I watched the birds build their nests and observed when the females joined. That spring, I learned what baby bluebirds sound like. Trying to write a podcast episode on my porch one afternoon, I kept hearing intermittent squeaks. When I looked up, I noticed they sounded each time a parent bluebird landed at their nest's doorway and delivered food. Each baby was saying, "Meeeeeeeeeeeee!"

Coincidentally (or not!), I chose the word *nest* a few months earlier as my business word of the year. I woke up a few nights in a row that January mumbling *nest* and decided it was there for a reason. Before we learned about COVID, I assumed my call to *nest* was to help me feel more permission to see fewer clients. My children were older school age at the time, yet I felt more maternal than when they were babies. I wanted to be a part of their activities. I wanted to be home when they got home from school (probably with store-bought cookies, though) and not stressed from a day of back-to-back clients.

That January I started to make my home reflect how I wanted to feel there; I brought in more plants, cozy blankets, and essential oil diffusers. I put up pictures and artwork that brought me pleasure.

As February turned to March, I remember connecting with how grounded and safe home felt for me. When we learned about the pandemic and that each time away from home was a risk, I felt grateful to come home to this respite. Standing masked and six feet apart from others at a grocery store, I often found myself crying. I could feel all the burdens we were carrying and the risks people working at the grocery store were making just to keep us fed. Coming home and sitting on my porch felt like the bluebird's nest: a reliable constant that protected me and helped me recharge safely.

We need more respite

Matilda sat down on my green office couch, noticed with a smile the white blooming tree outside the window, and let out a deep sigh of relief. It was audible and I could see her shoulders soften.

"It's good to see you, Matilda, and I notice the big sigh. What did you just let out?"

"There's something about this room. When I sit down here, I feel so much more at ease, even though we are about to do some hard work and I will probably cry. There's something about how I feel here versus the rest of the world. After each meeting I feel ready to take on whatever... yet that doesn't last. Maybe it lasts a few days, but then the real world sets back in and makes me put all my walls back up."

Once I moved a vase holding pencils in my office from the little table next to my chair to the mini dining table. Not thinking it was a big deal, my clients vocalized how alarming this was to them. Client after client, they all noticed the vase moving within seconds of walking in.

When I asked why they had noticed this, my clients said something along the lines of how the office layout was seared into their memory. They used it to help remember strategies and ways to implement them. The green couch and its surroundings offered a visual calm, reminding them they deserved to find their Food Voice. They carried that calmness the first few days after sessions, just like Matilda, yet usually it started to wane. When the disconnection inevitably occurred, visualizing the space and how one felt in it kept it a little bit closer. Clients said this helped them continue moving forward even when the diet industry and other oppressive systems tightened their grip.

After Matilda explained her experience in my therapy room, I found myself connecting the dots: we have so little opportunity to experience relationships and food discussions outside of the diet industry's influence. When we find something close (I can't claim my office space is free of diet culture and other oppressive systems but I certainly aim for it to be), we can dig deeper and do healing work. Sadly, that amounted to only one hour a week; sometimes clients saw a therapist, too, so we could add another hour. But what about the other 166 hours each week? How can we add more respite time?

Like the bluebirds, my clients built a part of their nest each time they met in my office. As they unpacked each script and met themselves with compassion, they noticed the traffic outside my window, the way the door chimed when someone entered the waiting room, or how the pencils were held tightly in a vase on my side table, not the kitchen table. Safety intertwined with these visual cues as they unpacked their complicated food history.

I imagine how, as you read this, you, too, are building a nest of thoughts, visuals, or other connections to the healing work.

I am grateful clients taught me how important this nest was to their forward-moving recovery of their Food Voice. I never moved a vase again! My clients taught me a valuable lesson (again): we need to add as much nesting time as possible to expand access to our Food Voice.

Adding more safer spaces gives you opportunities to understand what you need in your relationship with food and help you mend it. This chapter explores different ways to *nest* to help you rediscover and stay connected to your Food Voice, even when the outside world screams so loudly it's hard to hear. I encourage you to take this chapter as a brainstorm to get you building your own nest. It will help you stay connected to your Food Voice and out of the Diet Trap, promote health, and help set others free.

How to know if you need Nest Time

Your body will give you signs when you need to increase your Nest Time. I knew clients who came into sessions feeling disconnected from their body—whether it was signals they relied on to eat or values that guided their decisions—they needed more Nest Time. You may feel anxious, unhinged, burned out, or checked out. When you get these signs, you are not failing. You are not doing anything wrong, rather it is a sign that the world is still wrong. You are mending your relationship with food while on empty.

If you feel activated by a certain food choice or notice diet trauma, Nest Time can help. It recharges your supports and refuels your ability to tend to your complicated food history. Finding your Food Voice requires you to mend the past harms while still encountering punishment. Building literal and figurative nesting spaces carves out an opportunity to safely rest and heal even if just for a moment.

Daily Nest Time is a necessity to finding your Food Voice. Everyone needs it as long as the diet industry exists. How long you need it will ultimately come from your unique lived experiences and the oppressive systems pushing you toward your scripts.

Nesting spaces

"You look so great!" I heard this two weeks after giving birth to my oldest. Exhausted and probably smelly, I was so in love with my baby and shocked when this friend mentioned my appearance *first*. Not how kickass I was to push this baby out. No acknowledgment of my powering through my obvious sleep deprivation. And, most importantly, no acknowledgment of this new human who had come into existence.

Have you witnessed this phenomenon, too? People love to tell pregnant people and those postpartum how great they look. I hear this happens because it is what I should want to hear and because people are just being polite.

Speechless in these postpartum exchanges, I just said, "Oh."

If you think that is rude, that is okay. I was told it was, too. I could also feel the tension as the compliment-paying friend paused and waited to hear my thank you, but I couldn't comply. They never got it because I decided my home would be a safe haven from the diet industry. I was too exhausted to explain my one-word exclamation and decided *oh* was a full enough sentence just like *no*.

Just a few years later, I met Marilyn Wann, fat activist, at a Binge Eating Disorder Association conference. As I chatted with her, she offered me a printed half sheet of paper that read: *Welcome! Weight diversity is celebrated here. Kindly refrain from diet talk, body disparagement, and other unpleasantries. Thank you!*

I proudly posted it in the part of my kitchen where everyone walked past. This small sheet reinforced my nest. It didn't eliminate all food and body talk, but posting quickly stopped much of it. As my kids started eating table food and being a part of meal times, visitors brought their bad food and body talk. All I had to do was point to Marilyn's sign and folks would shut up.

As I moved to packing school lunches, preparing Thanksgiving turkey, and making grocery lists, I just had to look at the sign to remind me of my anti-diet values and my inherent worth outside of my appearance. This strengthened my Food Voice access and shielded people I loved from learning more about diet culture. I knew they would learn the diet industry's tools eventually, yet I wanted them to build a foundation for their food history without its influence.

We live in a world with an always-present diet industry; we need breaks from it, especially while finding our Food Voice. My home is my primary nest: a place I can always go back to where I can control the variables to keep me grounded, accepted, and unguarded.

Visuals, sounds, and scents provide this sanctuary. What could you visually add to your living space to give advanced permission to yourself? What could you add to help affirm those with different identities from your own to whom you are an ally?

While I am a visual person, clients have taught me other ways they have transformed their home to make it their nest. Consider adding scents from candles or essential oils that give you the feeling you want while feeling safer. Clients often spoke about how certain pieces of music or meditations have helped whereas others claimed that soft textures or weighted blankets did the trick.

What can you add to your home to help you and your brain know you are safer there? That this is a place devoid of the diet industry's influence and where your Food Voice is welcome to take up as much space as it needs?

When home can't be your nest

Matilda rolled her eyes when I mentioned building a nest within her home. "Have you seen where I live, Julie? Have you been to my campus? Everyone is trying to avoid looking like me. I am literally their worst nightmare."

She was correct: Matilda attended a college full of the thin, white, able-bodied people obsessed with diet and exercise. From the calorie counts in the cafeteria, to the unaccommodating painful chairs in the lecture halls, to the always-dieting roommates, Matilda could not safely nest where she lived.

Do you experience this, too? Do you have family or roommates who constantly diet? Or, even worse, who disparage your body and food choices? Like Matilda, does your home include furniture designed to not include your body?

You deserve better. You deserve a safe and comfortable place to go back to each day. When Matilda and I discussed this, she decided to add more nesting opportunities into her sensory fields to help cue moments of safety and rest. Let's explore ones you could add, too.

Other nesting spaces

Matilda's grandmother communicated unconditional love and acceptance. Matilda fondly remembered how much her grandmother looked similar to her, especially her belly. While her grandmother was no longer alive, Matilda remembered how it felt to be in the same room with her. "I used to go to her home after school and my grandmother was the cliche: baking cookies as I got home. She always made sure I had enough." Matilda chose a few candles that reminded her of her grandmother: ones that smelled like fresh-baked cookies as well as ones she found that smelled like her grandmother's favorite perfume. Each day, when getting back from class, Matilda would close her bedroom door and light a candle. Before journaling—something she found important during Nest Time—she'd wait a few minutes for her room to fill up with the scent. "Just smelling the memories reminds me how beautiful my grandmother was and at the same time how beautiful she said I was. If I connect with her beauty and she looked like me, I have to be beautiful, too."

Where can you add safe spaces to your life? Consider adding cues using sights, sounds, and smells.

Music

Which music helps you feel cozy and provides respite? Give yourself three minutes to feel what you want to feel by listening to what moves you. Consider creating a playlist to extend your break. I love that we can put headphones on anywhere, close our eyes, and disconnect from diet culture. Need ideas? Try out this playlist I created for you. Go to FindYourFoodVoiceBook.com or library.johnmurraylearning.com to discover the Find Your Food Voice Playlist.

Your workspace

Workspaces are not typically known for their positive food messages. Consider adding notes in your desk drawer to remind yourself of your worth. Put up pictures where you can that can help you fantasize about being somewhere else that captures your cozy feeling. Feeling bold and want to create change there? In Chapter 10 we discuss ways to influence your workplace food and body culture.

Your dining space

Paul and his partner decided to add a special bouquet of flowers to their dinner table each week. They both liked how it helped remind them they deserved the pleasure and satisfaction from each eating opportunity. What can you add to your dinner table or wherever you eat? Clients have added fun napkins, special plates, and framed pictures of loved ones far away. Others have found adding permission for screens helps them to disconnect and reconnect with safety whereas others have found not using screens helps them feel safer. Let yourself decide what you need at your dining space, and I hope you are okay if the answer is not what is typical.

Outdoor spaces

During COVID quarantine and even now, my front porch helps me nest. What outdoor spaces, if any, give you space to reconnect with your Food Voice? Do you remember Elena who decided to pause gentle nutrition sessions until she was ready? Elena spoke to me about a special tree she passed some days walking home from work. If she went a little out of her way, a dirt path took her to it and the blue bench sitting underneath. The tree seemed to arch perfectly, providing respite from the hot sun and shelter when it rained. Sitting there became her favorite nesting spot after working with people obsessed with dieting. She would listen to music, make her grocery list, and text with friends. Just looking at it helped her brain feel calm. No one could see the power of that spot just by looking at it, but it became an extended part of her nest.

Nesting boundaries

I am proud of you doing the hard work mending your relationship with food while finding new ways to reject your scripts. The longer you do this work, the higher the likelihood that you will need boundaries to support you. How do you set boundaries around food and body topics? I hope this part of the book helps you gather more tools to help secure more Nest Time that actually feels like respite. Elizabeth Armstrong, a licensed professional counselor, shared with me that boundaries not only keep out what you don't want but also include what brings value to your life. Boundaries help you bring that closer to your reality.

Navigating life outside of your scripts will require you at some point to communicate your needs. This is necessary advocacy work for you and other Voice Finders. Have you noticed a bad food comment or a self-deprecating body-size "joke" and been unsure how to react? Give yourself permission to navigate the diet industry however you can.

Sometimes that will be firmly reacting to an anti-fat comment with your words, and other times that boundary will look like leaving the room silently. There is no best way to add boundaries to your life, and honestly, you should not have to do this part. You are the oppressed; the oppressor should be the one advocating for Nest Time. Until we together make this cultural shift, and we will, let's consider different boundaries for you to experiment with in your life.

Armstrong taught me there are three different types of boundary that provide a way to insert space and communicate needs. They include:

Silent boundaries

Silent boundaries can be easy to start, and might include walking away when someone makes a fat "joke" or that "oh" of mine after a friend commented on my postpartum body. You may be tricked into believing that silent boundaries are not enough but resist that perfectionism. You are surviving. Silent boundaries my clients love include proactively wearing headphones or changing the subject.

Zero-tolerance boundaries

Elena texted her cousin before a get together to let her know that she did not want any negative food or body talk. She let her cousin know beforehand that, if a negative food or body comment came up, she would leave.

This is a boundary you can give to your healthcare provider before meeting them, too. Use that electronic chart access and send an email stating: *I have been traumatized by the push to diet in the past. I do not want to discuss my body size, get weighed, or given foods to cut out. I do not want to consider diet options to treat my symptoms. I have tried them enough to know they don't work for me.* If you have access to healthcare choices, use these boundaries and stick to them. Your healthcare providers work for you!

Ongoing educational boundaries

The most exhausting boundary includes explaining to folks about your complicated food history and why you are not going to follow a diet. This is not a one-time statement rather something that needs to be repeated in order for this person to completely understand what it means. Many folks I speak with expect to do this taxing education with every bad body comment or diet reference. If you have the energy to do this, we appreciate you! Please know most burn out quickly doing all this free education. Armstrong notes that oftentimes we can do this type of boundary setting with just two people at a time.

Nesting activities

The first few months writing this book, people within the PCOS Power Community came together for Nest Time. I wanted to be around others fighting the diet industry while writing and people within the community wanted virtual space for connection. I invited folks to join to do whatever they needed to help them mend their Food Voice in that moment. We called them *nesting activities*. I invite you to explore activities to mend your food relationship within your own personal nesting space and the community that affirms it.

Food planning

What comes to mind with the phrase *meal planning*? Do you picture pretty bento boxes with colorful combinations of fruits, veggies, and lean proteins? Do you get the message that meal planning is all about making sure you don't eat too much? Or that you shouldn't stray from the plan? Or, God forbid, that you shouldn't eat anything yummy?

Let's turn meal planning onto its head. Meal planning and preparing can be tools to ensure you have what you need on hand to stay disconnected from the Diet Trap. I want us to reclaim meal planning from diet pushers and weight-loss fanatics. Anti-diet meal planning and preparing can be a way to ensure you:

- have *enough* to eat
- have *satisfaction* with your meals and snacks
- avoid panic hunger.

Nest Time includes time to think about the necessary self-care that comes with nourishing yourself. If you had been following *I-Should-Eat* scripts for a long time, you depended on their ideas for food choices. You may have even used their products to be meal replacements. You may be surprised to learn how much time it takes to plan meals and snacks while finding your Food Voice. Over the years, clients have stumbled back into diets when they didn't carve out enough time to ensure they got enough to eat. Scripts strategically sell us ease with food; they plan our food structure so we don't have to make a decision. As you move away from your scripts, know making enough food will probably take longer than you anticipate. This doesn't mean you are too much of a burden or you are eating too much. Rather, this means you are recovering from your scripts and relearning what it takes to take care of your food and body.

It will take time to learn how to incorporate this type of self-care into your life. Here are some general guiding principles clients and I have incorporated. Know these are general and will depend on where you live, your access to foods, and their availability.

Monthly

What are your food staples? Are there cultural foods that make eating time complete? Certain foods you and your family rely on to make a meal? Elena knew she always had to have corn tortillas on hand because they were a part of every meal. Previous scripts tried to take them away as having too many carbs. When Elena discovered how much her body felt energized by fiber-rich foods, I reminded her that corn tortillas are an excellent source of fiber because corn is a whole grain. As Elena unpacked the racism that was trying to disconnect her from her cultural foods, joy returned to her eating experiences. "They feel like meals again!"

At first, Elena bought a small amount of tortillas to last the week, yet found herself often running out of them. This led to more unsatisfying meals and panic hunger. At one session, Elena and I brainstormed how to prevent this from happening. We considered a typical amount she needed per day and calculated how much she would need to get through a month. Just to be sure there was enough, we added a little extra to that total. Elena's favorite tortillas didn't last a month yet she found they kept great in the freezer.

Elena found this little bit of planning kept her from last-minute chaotic food experiences. She learned she could always throw together a complete meal at the last moment as long as she had tortillas.

What are your staples? What are things you can keep in your pantry or freezer to make meal and snack time easier? I encourage you to try to minimize the good versus bad thing here. Certain foods are frequent in your rotation for a reason. They may be cultural foods like Elena's tortillas or those easily accessible on your budget. They probably also taste delicious.

Every month, reserve 15 minutes of Nest Time to look over your staple food supply. Make a list of what needs to be replenished and add it to your weekly grocery list or order it online. Expect errors as you learn how much you need. Give yourself compassion as you figure this out.

Weekly

If you know me, you know I don't enjoy cooking. While this makes me a dietitian anomaly, I have accepted this long ago. Talking about food all day with clients, feeding myself, and feeding my children while not enjoying food preparation have their downside. My lack of cooking skills contributed to my lack of understanding of what I needed to have on hand to get through the week. While my children were young, I tried to plan weekly meals without regard to the actual schedule. I always worked late Wednesdays, yet would accidentally plan a multistep recipe that took an hour in the oven. I would arrive home from work, exhausted from my day, with kids wanting my attention, and have to spend over an hour in the kitchen. I lost count of the times I made this mistake before I committed to helping future Julie and making Wednesday an easy dinner night.

For me, pulling an already prepared frozen meal bought at the grocery store helped me survive along with my special *Hodgepodge Night.* This is where I would pull out clean cupcake baking trays and fill each one with different foods—nuts, string cheese, strawberries, Triscuits, celery slices, and olives. The kids would never touch the olives and mostly eat the string cheese and crackers with some nibbles on the rest. Hodgepodge Night was my way of cleaning out the fridge; sometimes I ate from the cupcake trays and sometimes I also added other leftovers that I would heat up just for me. Whenever I announced it was a Hodgepodge Night, my kids would squeal with delight. I always thought this was funny because it was the easiest meal to prepare.

It took me years to figure out a system to help manage how much food I needed at home and when to fit in grocery shopping days.

I eventually learned that, since I worked late on Wednesdays, I needed a slower Thursday morning to recover. After getting the kids to school, I set a two-hour boundary where I would not schedule clients or other meetings. I put on some reality TV I'd saved to watch, made some coffee to be drunk while still hot, and made my weekly grocery shopping list. The night before I probably started to notice what was needed as I cleaned out the remaining fresh food for Hodgepodge Night. I used to squeeze in a grocery run during this two-hour window yet eventually found the magic of online grocery shopping. I put the order in during this time, still drinking my hot coffee and enjoying reality TV. I would pick it up as I drove home from the office that afternoon.

Nest Time includes weekly meal planning for the week. Try to find a consistent pocket of time to look over your personal, work, and family (if needed) schedule. If there are any days where events take place during a meal time, pick an easy-to-prepare meal using shelf-stable or frozen foods—or plan to get takeout. Your future self will be grateful you already made the decision. If you are like me and misjudge how much you can do on these busy days, try to give yourself compassion and note what would have made it easier.

While making your grocery list, plan more than just dinners. How many breakfast meals do you need to have on hand? What do you need to be sure you have enough at lunch? Which snacks are you into?

Some advice: even if you think you will have plenty of time to prepare meals and snacks throughout the week, be sure to come home from the grocery store with at least one very easy-to-prepare meal. I always grab a frozen pasta of some sort—usually macaroni and cheese—since everyone enjoys that in my house. I always use it. I can just pop it into the oven or microwave, cut up some raw celery or plop baby carrots into a bowl, and add a side of grapes. *Voilà!* It's a meal.

Daily

Plans change, and your meal plan may need to change with it. Before you go to bed at night or in the morning, look at what you have going on that day. Consider what you planned for meals and snacks. Do you need to defrost anything? Can you chop anything now to make things easier for your future self after work? Did your schedule get all twisted up again and you need to change your dinner plans to take out?

Try to include 15 minutes of Nest Time at the start and/or end of the day to take care of your food planning needs. This will set you up to have enough and help you avoid panic hunger. If you find yourself constantly thinking about food outside of meal and snack time, this is a great sign you need more meal planning Nest Time. Working toward monthly, weekly, and daily Nest Time devoted to your food self-care will help your brain think about food less often. With all that is going on in this world, we need you fed and awake. Nest Time helps you reject the oppressive systems that keep the diet industry strong.

Food journaling without shame

Just like meal planning, food journaling tends to bring up rigid relationships with food and lots of shame. What if, instead of keeping track of calories, macros, or points, your food journal helped you figure out what self-care you need around taking care of your food and body?

I encourage you to explore a food record practice that notices topics like these:

- how satisfying or not a meal experience is for you
- CHIP feedback when a meal is exceptionally not filling or leads to a sleepy afternoon
- how stress or sleep impacts your food cravings
- when you accidentally skip a CHIP or don't have access, how this affects the day or week
- the microaggressions you experience and how they impact your Food Voice
- Curious Nutrition observations and all their nuances
- post dietitian, coaching, or therapy debrief to help you better retain all of the sessions' content
- any gratitude for the moment and wishes for the future.

If keeping any record about your food intake and movement activates a past experience or fear, I encourage you to compassionately notice it. It is okay to never journal again. It is also okay to rewrite how you journal to suit your mended food history.

Nest grounding exercises

The diet industry and its associated oppressive systems demand us to analyze and stay in our thoughts rather than in the present. I am prone to chronic anxiety; grounding exercises (along with years of psychotherapy and medication) unhook me from my magnetic anxious downward spiral. Especially if your scripts pull you into anxious thoughts, grounding exercises can kindly bring you back to where you want to be in the present, making your own decisions.

Experiment with grounding exercises to create Nest Time anytime and anywhere. Paul found silent meditation to be his favorite way to ground at the end of the day. He kept it simple doing the four-square breathing exercise:

1 Take a deep breath in for four counts.
2 Gently hold for four counts.
3 Let it out for four counts.
4 Gently hold for four counts.

Repeat four times.

He loved its simplicity and found his sleep to be more restful. "I don't have to worry about pulling out my phone which just sucks me into scrolling social media or checking email. That right there is half the battle. The breathing tends to slowly calm my self-talk and get me ready to rest." As he practiced this nightly Nest Time, he found he could use the four-square breathing exercise anytime throughout the day. "I can picture a square and go through the steps while waiting for court to begin, at a red light, or before a stressful meeting. I love that I can bring my nest anywhere now."

Meditation helps lower blood pressure and blood sugar and increase wellbeing.[1] What I like about meditation is that it requires zero equipment and can be done anywhere without anyone knowing it. You can create a nest within your brain to get back the present and remember how ill-fitting diets are to the life you want to create. Many clients used silent meditation at a daily consistent time whereas others just reached for it when they needed it. I trust you will find what fits best for you, including not including meditation as a useful grounding tool.

If you find your thoughts bounce around and silent meditation does not feel calming, consider experimenting with guided imagery. This type of meditation allows you to listen to someone describe places, feelings, or messages. In this digital age we can connect with hundreds of choices on apps like *Insight Timer* and *Calm*.

Want to try guided imagery designed to help you find your Food Voice? Go to FindYourFoodVoiceBook.com or library. johnmurraylearning.com for ones I have created for you.

Rae found that sitting and meditating did not fit for them. Rather, they felt fidgety and uncomfortable, which just made the script messaging loud. For Rae, slowly walking around their block, with no music, calmed their brain. They would notice the sights—how neighbors decorated their front doors and the status of the trees—and sounds—the wind rustling the branches and the types of bird chirping. "I find walking and just noticing helps my brain quiet. It's like I pick my nest up and float it around like a magic carpet observing the world."

While this type of grounding exercise was easy to access, weather often prevented it from happening. Very hot weather tended to make Rae nauseous and light-headed, and they lived in the Southern part of the United States where it felt hot from May through September. Rae found a secondhand under-the-desk walking pad for those days. Unlike treadmills meant to be sprinted on, this walking pad could only handle a gentle stroll. It tended to mimic the outside walk that grounded Rae. They positioned it toward a window and played the music they needed to ground in that moment.

Even if different meditations don't suit you, I still encourage you to explore ways to ground yourself. This could be as simple as stepping outside for two minutes between meetings to feel the ground under your feet. It could be stomping your feet on the ground after a long drive or flight. Open a window to feel the breeze or notice trees moving with the invisible wind. Put your hand on your heart and feel your chest move with a breath or two. Even if it feels awkward, letting your brain quiet and empty for a second will help you continue to mend your Food Voice. You can even imagine grabbing your Magic Wand from Chapter 3 and invest in that Food Voice reconnection.

Nest art

I gravitate toward creative people. Watching artistic friends create something from nothing helps me minimize the perfectionism that gets in the way of accessing my own creative side. Even if you are like me and feel "not good at" art, still consider adding it to your Nest Time. Adding creative endeavors to your Nest Time gives you an opportunity to disconnect or even dissociate. Letting your mind check out for moments every day gives you a break which will help you destress and bring clarity to your Food Voice.

I am determined to explore more creative pursuits in my life and challenge the perfectionism that is in my way. Typing these very words has been a big push to show me that I can withstand the mind trolls poking sticks at my self-esteem. Writing has become a grounding activity and providing more pleasure than I thought it would. Could writing be a new nest activity for you?

While writing may not be your thing, consider exploring these popular nest activities:

- coloring or painting
- scribbling
- crocheting, knitting, or sewing
- jewelry making or working on your Voice Finder Cord
- playing a musical instrument
- playing a video game
- putting on makeup or doing nails
- cultural crafts
- tinkering with an object to learn how it works
- puzzles.

What did I miss? What could you add to your nest time that helps you ground, recharge, challenge, or lose track of time?

Nesting people

Who supports you while you are mending your complicated food relationship? Many people start finding their Food Voice on their own, yet they need supportive people to keep going. How about you? Rejecting your *I-Should-Eat* scripts with every food decision without support will be isolating. Add as many people as you can while finding your Food Voice. Here are common options.

Professional

I wish our world normalized seeking mental health support, not just physical health services. You may have gone to the doctor for a regular checkup or when ill; do you do the same when your mental health needs attention? Those of us who have worked with a therapist or another mental health professional, let's name this in public to help destigmatize the experience. I remember the first time I heard someone admit to working with a therapist; it helped me visualize that as an option for me while in the throes of a depressive episode.

Professional support will provide more nesting options, yet do know not everyone deserves to be a part of your nest. Be selective if you have access to choices. Look for helpers with backgrounds in weight-inclusive care and non-diet tools, or who describe themselves as fat positive. Some professionals that could be a part of your support team include:

- registered dietitians
- mental health counselors
- psychologists
- social workers
- marriage and family therapists
- somatic experience practitioners
- movement or exercise trainers
- coaches.

Many clinicians will not agree with my recommendation to work with a coach. Coaches typically have a lower barrier to entry and less training and can often be more easily accessed. That quicker path to seeing clients is why I insist on including coaches here. All the other helpers listed require expensive, exclusive training that prevents diverse folks from completing the training. Completing requirements when you are Black, queer, disabled, higher-weight, or another historically marginalized identity can be dangerous or made impossible. It is important to have professional support from folks with a similar lived experience; working with a coach may be the way for you to experience this.

A common way for folks to recover from an eating disorder or the diet industry includes weekly sessions with different professionals. When clients worked with me as their dietitian, they also worked with a coach or mental health provider. I encourage you to try to schedule these meetings on different days and days apart if possible. For example, see your dietitian on a Monday and therapist on a Thursday. I have noticed over the years that momentum builds during sessions and can last a few days before it wanes. As it wanes, you can meet with the next person on your team to help build your mojo back up.

Peer or community

You are not alone rejecting your scripts yet I know the world makes it appear that way. Voice Finders like you will feel isolated, which can be a fast track back to the shame-and-blame script experiences. Seek out support groups and other ways to meet fellow Voice Finders. When I first started helping people mend their complicated food history, we had only "baby" Google and social media was just a twinkle in someone's eye. Local clients in my small town found it tough to find peers on the journey and often had to drive hours away for meetups. Even more, the chances of meeting someone they knew in real life was often too risky for someone to even seek peer support.

I want you to know that meeting with others with your lived experience navigating the diet industry will help you more than any book. It may even help more than any professional. I appreciate I can write words to help unlock your worth from your complicated food history, but that is not enough. Connecting with someone who shares your identities and is a few steps ahead can give you a glimpse of the path moving forward. Even more, you doing the same with someone a few steps behind you will fuel your journey and keep you out of isolating shame.

We live in a world that tells us to be productive, courtesy of capitalism's oppressive system. You've done so much already to examine your complicated food history. It is normal and natural to need rest. I encourage you to let go of expectations while finding your Food Voice and budget in more Nest Time than you think you need. In the end, you will probably need more than you estimated. This rest will be radical and strengthen you to help everyone reconnect to their own Food Voice.

Dear One Exhausted Human,

We have pulled up a comfortable supportive chair; please let yourself put all your burdens there and take a break. You deserve more from the world and we see you trying to access everyday things with a painful struggle. The world has tried so hard to isolate you, but know you are not alone. Indeed, others experience the same, and magic happens when you come together. This magic will fix the oppressive systems making us all sick. You see what so many others have yet to recognize; look to others on the same path even when they are hard to find. Keep looking for other Voice Finders with your identities. When you can't connect with them, offer yourself medicinal comfort and space with boundaries and rest. Because you carry more burdens than many others, you will need more care. Not because you are broken but because the world needs to be fixed.

Love,
Food

Dear Food letter activity

What if the whole world was a nest? Write a letter to Food describing your script-free utopia, one that never spoke the word *diet* and where the scale had as much meaning as a thermometer. What would chairs look like? What food would be served and how? How would we connect? Let your mind run wild and record it so we can manifest this.

Voice Finder Cord activity

Hold your cord and consider all of its parts. You have built a physical representation of your own unique Food Voice. Bring this with you at Nest Time or carry it with you throughout the day. Attach it to a bookmark and keep it in your journal. Clip it on your purse or backpack as a cue to stay connected or as armor when *I-Should-Eat* scripts predictably show back up.

You gave each knot and braid meaning. Meditate on each marker to reconnect with your intentions. Here is a reminder of each step in your Voice Finder Cord:

1. The first knot is your Voice Finder Knot symbolizing your unique relationship and history with food. Your Magic Wand guided imagery showed you a glimpse into your Food Voice, and this knot will help remind you of its constant presence. Even when you can't quite feel it, your Voice Finder Knot is always holding everything together.

2. The blue braid symbolizes Food Voice's flexibility. It reminds you:
   a. Food is morally neutral. It is neither good nor bad.
   b. My Food Voice does not have an absolute right or wrong next step in making my next food decision.
   c. When I struggle connecting with my Food Voice, I ask: How can I be flexible?

3. The green braid symbolizes Food Voice's kindness. It reminds you:
   a. My Food Voice prioritizes getting enough food.
   b. My Food Voice wants to offer one more in case I need it or want it.
   c. My Food Voice encourages me to eat more food to help me recover from when I was told I couldn't or shouldn't.
   d. When I struggle connecting with my Food Voice, I ask: What is the kind choice?

4. The purple braid symbolizes Food Voice's nurturing side. It reminds you:
   a. My Food Voice helps me cope with life.
   b. My Food Voice wants food for energy, pleasure, connection, and emotional regulation. All these wants make me a successful human.
   c. When I struggle connecting with my Food Voice, I ask: Am I nurturing my unmet needs?

5. Feel them all come together in the next knot.

6. Remember the next blue strand representing your past. This strand represents the food beliefs, customs, and experiences that your ancestors experienced. Some of these you may know and many you will not yet allow to live within you. Let your brain imagine their collective Food Voices and what they have wanted to pass down to you—whether those are helpful now or not.

7. Connect with the next green strand representing your present. What oppressive systems do you experience. Name them as you feel the braid. Recognize their massive power. Notice how you have been manipulated to not see them. See which systems you contribute to upholding and can change for the better.

8. Remember the next purple strand representing your future. What do you want to make different looking ahead? When you hold your Magic Wand and consider the possibilities, how do you want to relate to food? Your body? To movement? To others? As you feel the braid, repeat these future wishes and imagine them already complete.

9. This next knot combines your past, present, and future. It represents what is not yours: shame and blame. As you pass over this knot, say this out loud: *I-Should-Eat* scripts don't work for me because I am a successful human. This blame is no longer mine to carry.

10. Hold the blue family of string braided together next. This braid tells your *I-Should-Eat* script history. Gently rub this knot to remind yourself this is your data that scripts will not work for you. This does not make you a failure; it makes you a successfully evolved human.

11. Hold the green family of string braided together. This symbolizes your ongoing pivot away from your *I-Should-Eat* scripts. Stay grounded and ask yourself the six CHIP questions:
    a. Am I hot or cold?
    b. What am I feeling? Or if this fits better, what messages am I getting from my brain?
    c. Do I need to use the bathroom?

d. What are my thoughts focused on?
e. Am I physically hungry? How do I know?
f. Am I emotionally hungry? What does it symbolize?

12. Next, hold the purple string braided together. Consider which emotions, experiences, and messages you release. Some you know instantly reading this whereas others will emerge over time while you are finding your Food Voice. Gently rub the knot representing all those known and those still left unspoken. Honor their meaning then picture them all being gently carried away down a river.

Reference

1 Jamil, A., Gutlapalli, S. D., Ali, M., Oble, M. J. P., Sonia, S. N., George, S., Shahi, S. R., Ali, Z., Abaza, A., & Mohammed, L. (2023). Meditation and its mental and physical health benefits in 2023. *Cureus* 15(6). https://doi.org/10.7759/cureus.40650.

10

Speak

Dear Food,

. For as long as I can remember I've gotten mixed signals about how to have a relationship with you. I spent weekdays with my parents where you were restricted from me and weekends with my grandmother who showed love through you. I was a fat child. I can remember even as a toddler being ashamed of myself and refusing to have my picture taken.

The older I got the larger I became. I was alone a lot, and you were the only thing that was there for me. I abused you and I couldn't stop. The numb feeling you gave me seemed worth it at the time. The bullying got even worse in middle school and high school. I avoided everything and everyone. I get emotional to this day thinking about all the things I missed out on, things that "normal" kids and teenagers take for granted like going to dances, parties, and just being a kid. I spent most of my time lost in daydreams thinking, "If only I were thin I could do that."

During my sophomore year of high school, I quit you completely. I starved myself for a year and lost over one hundred pounds. I still wasn't happy. It was never enough for me, and I always felt like the fat girl. Over the next ten years, I was every size. I was obese, thin, average, and everything in between, over and over again.

Because I never learned how to love you. I decided the only thing to do is learn everything I could about you. I went to college to study nutrition to help myself and help other people avoid the sad and lonely years I endured. I learned how you nourish me, the incredible way you help my body function, and how to help others.

I have finally, after many years, realized that I will never be skinny. I'm in a slightly larger-than-average body now, and I'm finally learning that what I look like does not define who I am as a person. None of us is perfect, and loving oneself is the true way to peace and happiness. I don't want to miss out on anything else.

There is one thing I can't understand. When I tell people I am a nutrition major, I see the looks of judgment they give me. It's gotten to the point where I don't want to tell people. I have even been called a hypocrite, and sometimes I feel that I am. There are still times when I'm alone and use you to numb my problems. As an adult, I still get reminded that I'm not thin. I wish people knew the power of words and could feel the hurt it brings me. It takes me back to what I felt like as a child. I am graduating soon and fear what I will have to face when I'm in the food and health industry. How do I deal with this constant judgment, and how can you and I just exist in peace?

Love,
Me

A group of queer Black body liberation activists named diet industry harm back in the 1960s. They tried to stop the diet industry's increasing power in North America.[1] While many have never learned about this part of history, coming together decades ago started a ripple effect promoting legislative change, as happened in New York City.

"No one should ever be discriminated against based on their height and weight. We all deserve the same access to employment, housing, and public accommodations, regardless of our appearance," said New York City Mayor Eric Adams after passing Introduction Bill 209—banning discrimination based on height and weight—in 2023.

Do those 1960s organizers know about the NYC law banning height and weight discrimination? Did they ever get to see the change they started?

This chapter outlines ways you can advocate for yourself and your loved ones. You will find ways to start conversations, give ideas, or provide new structures. Just like the activists from decades past, know your work using your Food Voice will create a long-term powerful ripple effect. You may never know the seeds you plant, yet I hope that sets a fire fueling you to speak up when you can.

Healthcare

I hope finding your Food Voice changes the way you relate weight to health. I picture you lifting off that heavy shackle as you recognize the empty promises of permanent health and weight maintenance. If you have been trying to lose weight, you probably have had to perform at each healthcare visit: swearing you will adhere to the doctor's diet recommendations (even as they change and despite their not being rooted in evidence) and will try to try harder. I know you self-abandon in those moments because you are just trying to access medical care.

Something I want you to know: you should have access to equitable and comprehensive healthcare at every visit. I dream of healthcare that is accessible and full of ease for you, no matter your

- size
- gender identity
- blood sugar readings
- ability
- race
- language
- or other identities making healthcare inaccessible or unsafe.

As you sever your beliefs regarding weight and health, the healthcare industry still hasn't. I want to help you advocate for your needs while trying to navigate healthcare settings. You have permission to choose what, if anything, you'd like to take from this to your healthcare provider. I hope it provides organization, education, and information to get the most out of your meetings with them.

Preparing for your visit

Raise your hand if you have visited a healthcare provider, and remember a chief concern or prominent medical history only at the end of the visit. Even though I have spent years working in hospitals and doctors' offices, this routinely happens to me.

I encourage you to keep track of your medical history, description of diagnosis, date diagnosed or identified, who identified it, and how it was diagnosed. My clients have used a chart like this one, and it helps ease worries and prevent that *oh-shit-I-forgot-to-tell-you-something* at the end of the visit.

Personal medical history

Diagnosis	Date Diagnosed	Provider Name	How Diagnosed

Want your own copy of this chart? Go to FindYourFoodVoiceBook.com or library.johnmurraylearning.com.

Brainstorm questions for your doctor

Let's take some time to think of all the questions you have for your healthcare provider and write them down. That way, you won't forget when you're at the appointment. Think about symptoms that you've been experiencing, especially anything that has changed since your last appointment, or anything you want to know about different labs, medications, supplements, or symptom management options.

Want sample questions? Here are a few that my clients and I have put together over the years.

- **General**
  - I think about food and worry about it most of the day. Can you help me find a mental health provider that can help me without shaming me?
  - I regularly experience migraines. Is this related to any of my chronic conditions, and if so, do you have any suggestions?
  - What can I expect my cycles to be like after menopause?
- **Sleep and energy**
  - Regardless of how much I sleep, I don't feel rested when I wake up. Do you think it would be appropriate for me to get a sleep study done?
  - My energy levels feel low throughout the day. Do you have suggestions for how to improve them?
- **Insulin resistance**
  - Are there any new medications to help with my insulin levels?
  - Is there a way to measure my insulin levels beyond just testing my A1c levels?

- **Medications**
  - o What is the right combination of medications and supplements to manage my specific symptoms?
  - o My current medication has been making me sick. Are there any alternatives?
- **Fertility**
  - o What are suggestions that you have for me to manage my chronic disease symptoms if I don't want to have biological children?
  - o What are options that will help me when trying to conceive?

After making your list, I encourage you to prioritize your questions to the top three to five. Bring them already written in a notebook.

Setting boundaries with your doctor

I used to cower when confronting a doctor, but over time I have gotten better at it. I appreciate my experience in a smaller white body is not the same as those in more marginalized bodies, and I want you to know I am on your side.

Preparing mantras, prompts, or printouts has helped many people with a complicated history with food set boundaries with their healthcare providers. For more assistance and affirmation, I recommend the following folks for free and paid resources:

- Glenys Oyston (DareToNotDiet.com)
- Ragen Chastain (DancesWithFat.com)
- Lindley Ashline (BodyLiberationPhotos.com)
- Laura Burns (RadicalBodyLove.com)
- Deb Burgard (BodyPositive.com)
- Beth Rosen (BethRosenRD.com)
- Christyna Johnson (EncouragingNutrition.com)
- Vinny Welsby (FierceFatty.com).

Please keep this in mind: it is okay if you choose not to advocate for better care. Weight stigma and other oppressive systems are real and powerful. You should not have to stand up to the oppressor—it is the healthcare system's responsibility to stop discriminating.

You may find times when you are more confident than others. Some folks have reported feeling more confident when they have role-played the healthcare advocacy conversation with a trusted friend, family member, or therapist. If this is not accessible to you, folks have benefited from practicing that conversation in front of a mirror instead.

When you have the energy to advocate for yourself while navigating healthcare, consider these five additions to your Voice Finder advocacy toolbox:

1 **You don't have to be weighed.** I know lots of people who feel so much better about their health and body image when they don't know exactly what they weigh. Do you? Most US healthcare providers weigh patients to bill insurance. In order to successfully get reimbursed for the visit, providers provide three assessment measures. Do you remember what you do when you first get called in from the waiting room? You get weighed, your blood pressure taken, and your temperature read. Here's a secret: You can say you don't want to be weighed. You might have to educate the technician to write in "refused" in the chart yet this still counts for them when submitting for reimbursement.

2 **"I am in eating disorder recovery, so please hold the weight loss talk … It can literally kill me."** Eating disorders have the second highest mortality rate of all mental illnesses, pushing healthcare providers to be more likely to respect your boundary. Not everyone understands pursuing weight loss is the number-one way a person relapses in an eating disorder, no matter what they weigh. If you have *ever* experienced an eating disorder, this prompt could be lifesaving. Consider communicating the boundary this way: "I have battled a lifelong and serious life-threatening eating disorder. Pursuing weight loss always makes me relapse and gain more weight. I would love for you to suggest other suggestions besides weight loss to treat my health."

3 **Diets just don't work for me, so *what* else do you have?** Many people I know at diet rock bottom have dieted their whole life. How about you? If that is the case, why would a diet suddenly start to work? When a healthcare provider suggests another diet, consider responding with a statement Ragen Chastain wrote on her *Dances with Fat* blog: "I have been prescribed diets my whole life and they have never made me healthier, thinner, or happier. My research says this is typical. What else can you recommend?"

4 **What do you recommend to your thin patients to promote health?** Get used to this question. It is a great, efficient one. People of any size can experience every condition and disease. So how

can higher weight be the cause? This question helps rein in the healthcare provider and asks them to access the part of the brain they use when speaking to people in smaller bodies. The hope is that you will finally hear different information besides "Just lose weight."

5 **Do you love research? Ask for it.** Next time the doctor is treating you based on only your size, experiment with this (also from Ragen Chastain's blog): "I am really into researching my healthcare. Can you show me the study where the XYZ diet worked on people my size to both lower weight long-term and have a health benefit?" There is another, briefer way to ask this one from fat-positive psychologist Deb Burgard: "Show me the data!"

Your visit checklist

Let's prepare for the visit by packing comfort items, things to pass the time, and sustenance for support. I prepared this list hoping it helps you stay grounded or distracted—whichever you need while navigating healthcare.

water	☐
comforting snacks	☐
headphones	☐
your fully charged phone	☐
a book, magazine, or something else to do while in the waiting room	☐
pre- and post-visit journal prompts and guided meditations	☐
a note of the first day of your last period (if applicable)	☐
well-fitting robe and medical gown (your provider may allow you to bring your own medical gown. Laura Burns, my yoga teacher friend, taught me how Amazon and other websites have relatively affordable options through size 10X)	☐
a friend, family member, or trusted support person	☐
notebook and pen	☐
face mask	☐
personal ID	☐
insurance card (if applicable)	☐
list of your medications and supplements	☐
recording device, or voice memo app on your phone	☐

personal medical history ☐

visit recap form ☐

final, prioritized list of questions for doctor ☐

Consent for Weight-Inclusive Care document (see below) ☐

Emotionally preparing for your healthcare visit

How would you describe your past healthcare visit experiences? If they involved traumatic events, know your history is valid. If you avoid healthcare visits—whether you've been traumatized there or not—you are not doing anything wrong. You are trying to protect yourself, and that is your strength.

Healthcare should be a human right. Accessing healthcare while risking microaggressions is radical advocacy all on its own. You are taking risks that help others who come after you just by showing up. I hope you know that I see you doing this advocacy, and my clients have benefited from it already.

If you need extra support while navigating healthcare, let's get your needs met. I encourage you to notice what your brain and body messages are before your next healthcare visit. What thoughts, feelings, or messages are coming up for you? Consider these questions to get you to your specific pre-visit needs:

- How am I feeling or thinking in this moment in time?
- What is something I can do to release them?
- What is my biggest fear going into this appointment?
- How can I release that fear before going into this appointment?
- What is something that could help me feel relaxed and at peace with my visit?

I have prepared a guided meditation for you to help you prepare for your next healthcare appointment. Go to FindYourFoodVoiceBook.com or library.johnmurraylearning.com to download it.

Many Voice Finders report connecting with another person who is rejecting scripts helps ground and support them during healthcare visits. Rae ended up connecting with someone at an anti-diet support group and they texted each other before and after each healthcare visit. This friend also experienced diet trauma while seeking healthcare. Rae taught me how meaningful this support was for them to actually make appointments and get the care they needed.

I appreciate not everyone has access to someone who is rejecting the diet industry. If you feel isolated while finding your Food Voice, I encourage you to connect with fellow Voice Finders via social media, support groups, or meetups. Yes, there is a risk putting yourself out there, but you will be rewarded abundantly especially when you connect with people with similar lived experiences. There's only so much I can shine a light on with my lived experiences—something probably obvious as you are reading this. I appreciate my privilege and believe mutual shared lived experience to be the way to completely mend your Food Voice. You will find strength from your peers navigating these healthcare experiences. Even more, your peers will benefit from your presence. Witnessing your peers' need for support creates a radical advocacy loop lifting your voices up for more to be heard. Whenever you do this, please know I am grateful because this is where I see support making change for those most harmed by the diet industry.

During your visit

Let's set you up to get as many non-diet answers to your medical and mental health concerns. Consider asking your healthcare provider for the weight-inclusive care you need rather than the standard diet advice. Direct the healthcare provider staff to have it documented in your medical record. You can provide this information at check-in or when getting vitals. Some people email it to their provider before the visit. Be sure to ask your provider to place this information about your care in with your chart.

Need help? I have created a Consent for Weight-Inclusive Care document you can print off just for this purpose. Get your own copy at FindYourFoodVoiceBook.com or library.johnmurraylearning.com.

The first page is for you to fill out and use while accessing care. Check off what you need and fill in the spaces to make it your own. When printed double-sided, the flipside provides medical references for accessing care without weight loss and diets. While I can't promise it will guarantee weight-inclusive healthcare, it provides the rationale and resources that will hopefully plant an anti-diet seed.

I hope it helps make the visit more accessible! You may never know the impact, yet this worksheet has swayed many doctors as well as nurses, medical assistants, therapists, and front-desk workers. We need everyone on board to reject scripts. What's more, this may help them find their own Food Voice.

Consent for Weight-Inclusive Care

Thank you for seeing me today. I'm sharing this document because I'm choosing to explore healthy living without dieting or weighing myself. I have dieted for many years, and it's only brought on worse physical and mental health in the long run. Feeling like I will be judged for "failing" has also made it harder for me to seek needed medical care. Please know my choice does not mean I'm giving up or neglecting my health. It means I'm now pursuing evidence-based ways to manage my health that don't involve trying to lose weight.

Studies show that the majority of your patients will not be able to achieve or maintain weight loss and will feel stigmatized in the process. I know this reality must make patient care hard for you, too. If you'd like to explore this more, along with weight-inclusive approaches shown to enhance patient outcomes, please see the opposite side.

- **Here's what I ask of you during our visits:**

  - Please do not weigh me. I do not consent to being weighed unless absolutely medically necessary (going under anesthesia, medication dosing, monitoring fluid shifts, etc.).
  - Please don't recommend a diet or lifestyle change or promote weight loss in order to treat any medical conditions or otherwise promote wellness.
  - Please don't discuss cutting out a food group or macronutrient. Only suggest removing a particular food in the case of allergy or a medication interaction.
  - Other:

- **Here are the ways you can support me:**

  - Please offer ways to treat my medical conditions and general health without focusing on weight. Consider giving me the same direction you'd give someone in a thinner body.
  - Help me advocate for comprehensive healthcare. Because of my size, I am often not able to get adequate care. Weight discrimination prevents me from going to the doctor to avoid traumatic experiences. I know this harms my health.
  - Ask me about my eating and exercise habits before assuming I am eating too much or exercising too little.
  - Help me add foods rather than restricting certain foods. Do not label a food as good or bad.
  - Help me explore health and manage symptoms in my current body.
  - Other:

Thank you for your partnership in my health!

| _____ | _____ | _____ |
| (print name) | (signature) | (date) |

Why weight-inclusive approaches improve patient health

Healthcare currently prioritizes weight as a principal determinant of health, prescribing weight loss as a means to treat health problems. This approach wrongly assigns responsibility for health conditions to patient choices typically perceived as causing higher weight, and blames patients for their disease and for failing to lose weight.

In contrast, the growing movement toward weight-inclusiveness in healthcare offers professionals the means to critically evaluate the efficacy of weight-loss treatments and create realistic, individualized treatment options that reduce stigma and support patient wellbeing. Recommending weight-loss interventions can have drastic long-term implications such as eating disorders, avoiding medical care, and worsened health.

For a thorough overview of weight-inclusive care, including all supporting references, please see the 2014 article by Tracy L. Tylka and colleagues published in the *Journal of Obesity*.[2] To briefly summarize its findings:

Weight loss treatments are ineffective, especially long-term.

- Evidence shows that long-term weight loss is not sustainable for most people.
- No major medical weight-loss initiatives have generated long-term results for the majority of participants.
- Evidence reveals that environmental, socioeconomic, and genetic conditions outweigh voluntary actions in leading to higher weight.

Weight cycling is linked to adverse health outcomes.

- Major longitudinal studies, such as the Framingham Heart Study and the German EFFORT cohort, associate weight cycling with increased mortality and morbidity.
- Experimental studies show weight-loss programs disrupt metabolism, reducing energy expenditure and requiring fewer calories to maintain the same weight versus those who have not dieted.
- Weight cycling is linked with poor psychological outcomes, and dieting is associated with the onset and maintenance of eating disorders.

Weight-normative approaches create stigma and interfere with health seeking.

- Studies reveal that higher-weight patients experience weight bias from medical and psychological professionals, including from those who treat obesity and eating disorders.
- Weight stigma can be internalized and contribute to poor health practices and outcomes. If you are interested in learning more about weight discrimination and mortality, please reference this to begin: Angelina R Sutin, Yannick Stephan, and Antonio Terracciano, Weight Discrimination and Risk of Mortality, *Psychological Science* 26.11 (2015): 1803–11 (DOI 10.1177/0956797615601103).

Weight-inclusive approaches support the many factors involved in health and wellbeing.

What is the alternative? Weight-inclusive practices widen the lens beyond weight and recognize the many factors that support human health and wellbeing. Such practices critically review the evidence for weight loss treatments, resolve to do no harm, and incorporate a weight-inclusive model, such as Health at Every Size (HAES). They use multidimensional, evidence-based approaches to enhance health and wellbeing at any weight. Patients are supported through reduced weight stigma; effective treatments; increased autonomy, access, and participation; a focus on process over end goals; and an inclusive view that prioritizes wellbeing for all sizes.

Commonly requested labs and studies

Removing the scale as a healthcare measure opens up the opportunity
for you to get more holistic and concrete healthcare information.
Every week, people contact me to get ideas on which labs (laboratory
tests) to order or which studies to run. Here are my most common
recommendations.

Yearly Lab Requests

Test	Normal Range	Purpose And Common Directions
Blood sugar and insulin		We recommend monitoring insulin along with blood sugar. Tracking this will help you to get a picture of how your insulin levels are impacting symptoms and how close you are to diabetes.
HOMA-IR	<1 optimal >1.9 early IR >2.9 IR	Gives you a picture of how much insulin your body needs to make to keep blood sugar in a normal range. This test is designed to measure insulin resistance, an early stage of diabetes. Insulin resistance makes most people produce an abundance of insulin; this will make fasting blood sugar and A1c appear normal without giving a picture of metabolic health. This is calculated using a fasting insulin and fasting glucose level. You will need to stop eating before midnight for this test.
2-hour post-prandial BG (via OGTT)	<140 mg/dL	This test measures your blood sugar 2 hours after eating a meal. In the event a HOMA-IR is not available or accessible, this test helps to show how quickly the body can bring down glucose levels. With high circulating insulin levels along with insulin resistance, blood sugar will often normalize yet take longer to get to that point. Often folks will need to stop eating before midnight to take a fasting glucose, then consume a set amount of carbs for the post-prandial blood sugar level.

A1c	<5.6 normal 5.7–6.4 prediabetes >6.5 diabetes	A graduated average of your blood sugar over the last 90 days, this provides a snapshot of your blood sugar management. This does not measure for insulin resistance and can be skewed to look normal when insulin resistance is present. It will not matter if you have eaten prior to this test or not.
Fasting blood sugar	<126 mg/dL (diabetes) <110 mg/dL (prediabetes)	Track this value yearly to monitor any shift in diabetes trajectory. This does not capture insulin resistance. You will need to stop eating before midnight for this test.
Lipid panel		Metabolic consequences to PCOS, diabetes, and insulin resistance include high cholesterol. Monitor these labs yearly to follow trajectory and intervene as necessary.
Total cholesterol	<200 mg/dL	You will need to stop eating before midnight for this test
LDL	<100 mg/dL	The cholesterol that you want lower because it can promote heart disease. You will need to stop eating before midnight for this test.
HDL	>40 mg/dL	The cholesterol that you want higher because it helps prevent heart disease. You will need to stop eating before midnight for this test.
Triglycerides	<150 mg/dL	This lab often increases as blood sugar starts to increase (even if not tracked well with A1c or fasting blood sugar labs). You will need to stop eating before midnight for this test.
Androgens	Use to help your medical provider diagnose PCOS and monitor its treatment.	Track how your interventions are adjusting your androgen levels if you are wanting to lower them. Your doctor may ask you to get this lab work done in the morning. It depends on the doctor whether or not food is allowed up until test time.
Total testosterone	6.0–86 ng/dL	The amount of total testosterone, including free testosterone

Free testosterone	0.6–3.6 ng/mL	The amount of testosterone that is unbound and actually active in your body.
DHEA-S	35–430 mcg/dL	Androgen secreted by the adrenal gland.
Other		
Vitamin B_{12}	<200–900 ng/mL (low risk) 1-3 mg/L (moderate risk) >3 mg/L (high risk)	Metformin depletes Vitamin B_{12} absorption in the gut and requires supplementation. Check this lab before starting Metformin for a baseline and yearly. It will not matter if you have eaten prior to this test or not.
C-reactive protein	<1 mg/L	This measures for chronic inflammation. Inflammation can predict disease. Monitor inflammation trajectory with this test. It will not matter if you have eaten prior to this test or not.
25 hydroxy vitamin D	20–50 ng/mL	Low vitamin D levels can cause extreme fatigue, inflammation, and infertility. Prescribed supplementation is often required to normalize levels. It will not matter if you have eaten prior to this test or not.
TSH	0.45–4.5 uIU/mL	This lab provides a general snapshot into whether a more thorough thyroid panel is necessary. It will not matter if you have eaten prior to this test or not.
T3	24–39%	Regulates basic metabolic function. The "3" in the name represents the number of iodine atoms it has. It will not matter if you have eaten prior to this test or not.
T4	4.5–12.0 ug/dL	Regulates basic metabolic function. The "4" in the name represents the number of iodine atoms it has. It will not matter if you have eaten prior to this test or not.
Sleep study		Sleep studies can be completed in a sleep lab or done at home. Your doctor will provide more specific instructions.

After your healthcare visit

I hope you give yourself space to breathe after every healthcare encounter. You navigated a challenging space and witnessed oppressive systems in action. This raises blood pressure, insulin, and inflammation. When we experience this type of physiological stress, rest can serve you to counteract the harm. If possible, I encourage you to give yourself extra time to attend to your needs, meditate, nap, and receive support.

Emotionally recovering from your healthcare visits

What feels like support for you after navigating healthcare? Notice what your brain and body messages are after your visit. What thoughts, feelings, or messages are coming up for you? Consider these questions to get you to your specific pre-visit needs:

- What are three things I feel grateful for in this moment?
- How can I be patient with myself and show myself more grace?
- Name at least two reasons why I am grateful for scheduling this appointment and following through.
- What do I wish I said in the visit differently or said at all?
- What new questions, if any, have come up for me after this visit?
- Who can I connect with to help me with post-visit support?

I have a post-visit guided meditation for you. Go to FindYourFoodVoiceBook.com or library.johnmurraylearning.com to listen.

Managing healthcare information

Keeping track of your healthcare changes like medications and supplements can be a full-time job, especially if you have chronic conditions. I hope you find the following charts helpful while advocating for your healthcare needs.

Visit recap notes

Visit Highlights

Changes In Symptom Management

Personal Visit Reflections

Follow-Up Steps (From Doctor)

Follow-Up Steps (From You)

Track your care: medications

Medication	Dosage	Dosage + Frequency	Start Date	Notes

Track your care: supplements

Medication	Dosage	Dosage + Frequency	Start Date	Notes

Schools and other learning spaces

Do you remember Traci? She found pears triggered too much diet trauma to add them into her eating. Typically when Traci came to our weekly appointments, her mom, Keisha, would work on her laptop using my office WiFi. Traci and I had a routine where we would meet for 45 minutes, then I would go to the waiting room to bring her mom into the session for the last five minutes. Every time I came to get her for our session wrap-up meeting, Keisha was multitasking, talking on the phone and typing away on her laptop. As a fellow mom, I appreciated how she used that 45 minutes efficiently to take care of things while stuck in a waiting room.

On a particular day, Keisha changed the routine. Traci glared at her mom as Keisha requested to meet with me first. She reassured her daughter the switch-up did not mean she was in trouble yet it was about a school issue.

When I brought Keisha into my office and shut the door, I heard Keisha let out the biggest sigh and plop hard on my green sofa.

"Oooooh, I can tell something is up. How can I help?"

"I am so angry right now, so if I start raising my voice, please know it is not toward you. It's just that Traci and my whole family have been through the ringer helping her recover from this eating disorder. Every week for the last year, she has come to see you and her therapist, she has been kicking and screaming while increasing her meal plan, and had to miss out on teenage things while her body was trying to heal. Her brain is finally in a good place: she is laughing and going out with friends. She isn't as moody or weepy. I am so afraid that her school is going to mess it all up."

Keisha goes on to tell me about a new pilot program at her daughter's high school. Apparently, the school teamed up with a local university, and they are studying what happens when teens wear pedometers and learn how to count calories to match their output. The parent handout described the study's purpose—intervening to prevent late-teen-onset obesity.

Keisha filled me in on the details: Traci would be required to wear a pedometer and share the data (how many steps she took over a week) with her classmates. Then, Traci would need to keep a detailed food record—and this one felt like a big punch in my face—and calculate the calories. As a class, the students were going to share if they ate too much or not.

My face fell. This type of experiment could be deadly for Traci. She had already been counting calories for years and matching it to how much she "burned off" with exercise.

But Keisha and I had more than just Traci on our mind. How would this experiment affect her classmates? Who else was struggling with an eating disorder? Who had the genetic profile for an eating disorder that this activity might trigger? What about Traci's higher-weight peers? How would discussions on obesity and avoiding weight gain impact them? How would this experiment teach weight stigma as a good thing?

Keisha, a higher-weight person her whole life, shared those same fears. "Traci started her 'healthy eating' because of a health class discussing what to eat to prevent weight gain. I know Traci was scared to be fat like me and eating 'right' would keep her from looking like me. At first, I thought that was a great idea—I have experienced a lifetime of bullying and I wanted to protect her from that. It took me until Traci was in the emergency room because her heart rate was too low for me to see how wrong we were.

"As she started to recover, I read into how the diet industry triggered all this. I learned how diets don't work, and if they do, it is often because those dieting are also in the throes of an eating disorder. Searching online for help, I went down a rabbit hole that brought me to fat-positive websites and social media. Traci's eating disorder helped expose mine. It helped me understand my body has always been fat and will always be fat. And that is okay. This is me at my healthiest—and still fat. Traci is coming along, too! And this activity will set her back so much, and I know it will negatively impact all of her classmates. Can I just keep her out of school for the two weeks it is going on?"

As Keisha and I processed this information more, we saw in tiny print on the very bottom of the study's information sheet, a way to opt out of the study.

This was not good enough for Keisha. "We must do something."

We brought Traci back in the room to fill her in on what we discussed. From there, the three of us strategized how to intervene. Traci pulled out her school laptop, a fresh Google doc, and the three of us got to writing.

Over the last 20 years, I have seen hundreds of people triggered to start eating disorder behaviors because of what was taught to them about eating, movement, or body size at school. Common school-based eating disorder triggers included:

- health class units on nutrition requiring calorie counts
- cafeteria menus with red, yellow, or green marks to let students know which foods you should and should not eat. Many included calorie counts
- children getting detention or demerits, or getting scolded for bringing in "unhealthy" food to school
- children being forced to eat the "healthy" items in their lunch first
- school assemblies teaching with fun music and a mascot how to avoid child obesity and help their higher-weight peers make "smarter" choices.

If you, like Keisha, want to speak up, I appreciate you. This is tough work, yet it can impact hundreds of people.

The following are building blocks while crafting an advocacy letter to a school raising a concern about food, exercise, or body image. Feel free to use the exact language I use or change things around. Further, use all of the pointers or just the ones that make sense for you.

Part 1

Give a brief description of what alerted you to the matter. I encourage you to write this part so you can inform the school leadership on the basics, including the class, instructors, and dependents involved.

Part 2

I encourage you to lead in with a statement such as: "I appreciate and value health. All kids deserve access to enough healthy food and to learn how to take care of their body. While I want my kids to learn more ways to take care of themselves, teaching diets and anti-obesity campaigns harm schoolchildren."

Part 3

Why does teaching diets harm children? Consider each block below a possible bullet point for your letter. Pick and choose which you want or use them all. Even more, add the information I left out!

a Promoting diets teaches higher-weight bodies are bad. This increases weight stigma and weight-based bullying. Expect more bullying after this program. While I appreciate the goal of helping higher-weight children to be healthy, this type of presentation just keeps them isolated, depressed, and stigmatized. Stigmatization has been shown to increase blood pressure, cholesterol, and other markers of poor health. The very markers they are told they cause by their increased weight can be explained by their mistreatment. Teaching size diversity helps *all* kids move their body and eat more healthily. Imagine how you'd feel if you were a fat child reading that handout that says they are battling *you*?

b Jean Piaget, the psychologist who extensively researched child development, taught us most kids are concrete learners until age 11. Concrete learners rely on black-and-white rigid thought patterns to navigate the world. Teaching food moderation, an abstract nuanced topic, can be understood only by those advanced in their formal operational stages of thinking.

c Because young kids are concrete learners, the ones with anxiety, OCD, or something like this will *fear* foods that are "bad" or in "red light" categories. Because of the brain's immaturity, the only way they will understand the statement "Soda is bad" will be like "Hitting your brother is bad." They will think this is a moral failure and truly take it to heart. Many third to eighth graders start to succumb to an eating disorder after programs like this.

d   To me, this is serious not only because of the deadly harm it causes children and families generally, but because I am concerned for my own particular child. There is a strong family history for eating disorders; since I know they are genetic, I need to protect my child. The best protection is to be sure my child never diets. For someone with a genetic predisposition to eating disorders, going on a diet is much like a person with alcoholism in their family taking their first drink. My child does not know about this genetic predisposition yet, and I will tell her later in life, just not yet.

e   Those at genetic risk for an eating disorder get information in school assemblies and health classes to start practicing an eating disorder. Eating disorders have the second highest mortality rate of any mental illness, and the earlier they start, the harder it is to recover.

f   These nutrition lessons leave kids confused: their parents gave them these "bad" foods. Does that mean their parents don't love them, want them healthy, or keep them safe? They get these same foods as rewards, often at school. *They are getting a mixed message.*

g   This programming teaches kids to distrust their hunger and fullness cues. Disconnecting these hunger and fullness cues promotes negative body image and teaches the kids to not trust their instincts.

h   This type of programming teaches kids how to diet. Dieting predicts weight gain (surprising, I know!) and eating disorders, as well as poor school performance.

It is not just *me* that feels this way, and it is not that I do not keep up with weight science. The American Academy of Pediatrics, the Academy of Eating Disorders, the International Association of Eating Disorder Professionals, the Association of Size Diversity and Health, and many others are with me. I am happy to send resources that they have written on why.

Part 4

Let the school know you will only allow weight-inclusive education. Play around with how you want to write this, yet my clients and I have used this statement: "Moving forward, I require knowing when the next nutrition education of any kind will be delivered to my children; I will need to pull them out for their protection."

Part 5

Let the educator know you would be happy to sit down with them to explain this in more detail or provide more resources.

By the end of the session, Traci, Keisha, and I had crafted an email to send to Traci's school principal. She also copied in the health teacher in charge of coordinating the study. At first, the school replied by saying they were just teaching healthy eating and not singling out higher-weight kids. The health teacher also went on to say that weight gain was a big issue in her classes and being a part of this university's study could impact students forever.

Exactly. Keisha and I worried about the long-term harm. Keisha felt compelled to forward the dialogue to the school superintendent and arranged a meeting.

Other ways to use your Food Voice in schools

School food systems

The diet industry and other oppressive systems flourish in schools, too. Even if you don't have to intervene with negative food and body talk, your Food Voice impacts in other areas. Sixteen million kids experience hunger each year,[3] and the school cafeteria can be the unexpected hero. Are you thinking about an unappetizing visual representing common school cafeteria food? Something I know to be true: school cafeterias are grossly underfunded and still magically feed 43 percent of each student body.[4]

Finding your Food Voice honors impacts from oppressive systems including those keeping people stuck in poverty and other kinds of food insecurity. If you notice insufficient or unappealing food at your child's school, look into it first instead of just complaining. While underfunded, most school cafeterias have little support from staff and students.

I believe the cafeteria workers are underappreciated when it comes to taking care of our children.

There are many ways to support school cafeterias. Consider these ideas:

- Ask cafeteria staff what they need to have better working conditions.
- Can you volunteer your time to prepare or serve the meals to help understaffed cafeteria workers have better working conditions.
- The more kids utilizing school lunch, the more funding most school food programs get. If you can afford it, consider letting your child rely on school lunch as often as you can, too.
- The more kids that buy and eat school lunch, the less stigmatizing it will be.
- Teach your children to never negatively comment on school food. Teach them words like *disgusting* or *gross* are not okay. Your kids are bound to call your own food gross at some point! Let them know in age-appropriate language that using these negative words dehumanizes people and promotes discrimination. Instead, I recommend saying "No thank you" when not wanting a certain food or "It's not my favorite but you do you."
- Teach your kids to not bully kids eating food from the cafeteria or eating food that appears unusual. Even more, teach them to intervene when others are getting bullied for this. Many of my clients have told me that one peer speaking up has gone a long way.

Access issues

The world is built for able-bodied, thin people. If you are an able-bodied and thin parent or caregiver, remember trying to squeeze into the preschool-size chairs? This is what our higher-weight kids and peers experience every day at school.

Matilda's best friend, Cherie, observed Matilda wince when getting into their interior design lecture class chairs a few days in a row. Matilda told me that one day, while hanging out together, Cherie noticed the same thing happen at the library. It was just the two of them studying together, and Cherie gently asked whether she was in pain. Matilda explained to her friend about how almost all of the seats at their university were too small for her. Cherie listened to Matilda explain how tough it was to navigate their campus and basically never be comfortable. She showed Cherie the bruises on her hips, and Cherie's face fell. She got teary-eyed and said she didn't want her best friend to be in pain. Could she help?

From there, Cherie and Matilda set off together to make their campus seating more accessible. They first spoke to the librarian and professors about the seat issue. When they said they couldn't help, Matilda and Cherie went to the department chair. She knew who to speak to about this—vital to a campus community that preached its accessibility on campus tours.

Health curriculums

As a dietitian, I hope every school teaches nutrition. As an eating disorder dietitian, I fear every school that teaches nutrition. I have lost count of the clients whose eating disorder or chronic dieting history began after a school food lesson. As I mentioned while drafting the letter with Keisha and Traci, too many focus on teaching calorie counting, BMI, and good/bad food labeling, while promoting the thin ideal. They sadly also contribute to worsening weight-based bullying and discrimination.

If you have control over school food lessons or can intervene to change one at a school near you, consider these as alternatives:

- Gardening lessons teaching kids how food is grown. Let them "harvest" their seeds and sample them if they like. Share which nutrients humans get from those foods.
- Lessons on foods from around the world, teaching about ingredients students may never see and how to respect the cultural connections of food.
- Sharing a food your family enjoys so that the whole class can learn about each student's cultural foods.
- While sampling different foods, lead a discussion on how we know when we are hungry or full. Demonstrate language one could use just like we teach names for feelings. Use words/phrases like *panic hunger*, *meal hunger*, and *snack hunger*. Teach how to use a hunger and fullness guide as one way to *trust* the body's intuitive regulation of foods.
- Teach how to do CHIPs and include lessons on mindfulness, getting enough rest, and ways to disconnect when times feel stressful.

- Provide a size diversity history lesson. Demonstrate how there have always been fat and thin bodies as well as other ways in which humans are diverse. Add books with diverse bodies including diverse body sizes in the school library.
- Educate on the harms of weight-based bullying and teach how to intervene. It is always best to learn about weight stigma from someone who experiences it. If there is no one able to teach this lesson who experiences weight stigma, still teach it, yet learn how to teach this class from a higher-weight person.
- Teach the dangers of dieting and how to avoid diets.

Work spaces

Finding your Food Voice at work will be challenging. Workplace weight loss challenges hope to inspire health improvements yet rarely work. Many health insurance companies now include price incentives to those who have a lower BMI or participate in commercial weight-loss programs.

I hate how these are now normal. My disdain comes from the pain my clients shared when trapped in these situations. Higher-weight clients silently struggled to recover from anorexia nervosa, but no one noticed because of their body size. Every year, clients felt pressure to join another New Year Weight Loss Challenge, even though they know it could be a fatal decision. Others, years into recovery, relapsed after having to join WW because of their recovery's high (and necessary for recovery) BMI.

You deserve to take care of your body however you need while at work. The diet industry promises companies they will save money if their employees lose weight. They don't warn how this creates more eating disorder behaviors, triggers relapse, probably worsens long-term health, and reinforces weight stigma.

If you find yourself having to choose to participate in a company-wide health initiative, I encourage you to be compassionate with yourself no matter what step you choose. If you decide to go ahead and just check the box to participate so your boss stops bugging you and you encounter less weight-based discrimination, I am proud of you. You made the best decision for you. If you decide to push back and demand the lower insurance rate even without joining WW, I am rooting for you.

Want to roll up your sleeves and get to work changing your workplace? Thank you! Here are some facts ...

- We have more than a hundred years of research showing diets don't help most people improve health long-term. Research has shown this to be the case for worksite wellness programs, too.
- While many diets improve some health markers in the short term, diet research teaches us that they only worsen blood sugar, blood pressure, insulin, cardiovascular health, and energy levels.
- You can't tell by looking at someone if they have an eating disorder, and worksite wellness programs make it unsafe for those trying to recover. Eating disorders have the second highest mortality rate of any psychiatric illness, and dieting behavior can be deadly.
- Dieting behavior is the greatest predictor of an eating disorder. People in midlife can experience a new eating disorder, too, and I fear this wellness program will trigger new people to experience an eating disorder.
- Pushes for employees to lose weight or lower their BMI don't improve health and only promote discriminatory practices. Worksite wellness programs create more opportunities to discriminate against higher-weight colleagues. Not only is this discrimination morally wrong, it also harms people's health.

Over the years, my clients and I have come up with alternatives to workplace weight-loss programs. Consider these when offering alternatives:

- stress relief
- smoking cessation
- meditation
- hunger prevention and food security initiatives.

Voice Finders unite!

"It's not you. It's not me. It's all of us. Only together can we fix diet culture. And we will."

Introduction to the Find Your Food Voice podcast

You have done such hard work finding your Food Voice. You've gone through every page of this book, done each exercise, and taken the time to better understand your complicated food history.

I've sometimes fondly imagined a quick-start guide with just a few pictures that would get you up and running in five simple steps, with no need to read this bulky manual—get you started now without any heavy lifting. But do you know why there's no quick-start guide included in this book? Or why the work isn't done at the end of Chapter 10? We know non-diet living would be less complicated if it was just up to individual choices.

We desperately need systemic change to give everyone access to their Food Voice. The work you've done going through this book will contribute to your own relationship with food and at the same time help others find theirs.

There is a path forward that won't leave *anyone* behind. To get there, we must rally together to make finding your Food Voice simpler for those behind us. Working together is the only way to help break down oppressive systems blocking many from accessing a world without *I-Should-Eat* scripts.

There's something in it for you: helping others find their Food Voice helps you stay connected to your own.

Are you with me?

Dear Me,

The world has been cruel to you, and you deserved to learn how to take care of you lovingly, no matter your size. Now that you have been training to be a healthcare provider, you have a new set of tools. We see how hard it has been to survive this training: anti-fatness rooted in racism will do everything in its power to keep you from taking up space. Every time you reject that oppressive system—no matter how loudly and even if your voice shakes—you shatter miles of walls keeping another from their Food Voice. We are grateful you have been so brave, and we hope others will do the same for you. It is truly the only way we can move forward.

Love,
Food

Dear Food letter activity

Write a letter to Food describing how someone could have advocated for you. When do you wish someone else had spoken up? How would things be different? How can you use this past experience to promote change?

References

1 Griffin, M., Bailey, K. A., & Lopez, K. J. (2022). #BodyPositive? A critical exploration of the body positive movement within physical cultures taking an intersectionality approach. *Frontiers in Sports and Active Living* 4(908580). https://doi.org/10.3389/fspor.2022.908580.
2 Tylka, T. L., Annunziato, R. A., Burgard, D., Daníelsdóttir, S., Shuman, E., Davis, C., & Calogero, R. M. (2014). The weight-inclusive versus weight-normative approach to health: evaluating the evidence for prioritizing well-being over weight loss. *Journal of Obesity.* doi: 10.1155/2014/983495.
3 https://www.feedingac.org/ (accessed March 18, 2024).
4 https://schoolnutrition.org/about-school-meals/school-meal-statistics/ (accessed March 18, 2024).

Epilogue

Rally

Matilda

Matilda sat down on my green couch one last time. We knew this day was coming and it was certainly bittersweet. She had a new job teaching on the West Coast. She successfully defended her doctorate dissertation the week before on accessible interior design.

After Cherie and Matilda connected with their department chair, the university put in place campus-wide requirements for safe accessible seating in every classroom. This took two years to make happen, and Matilda had to meet with many different faculty members to get them to understand how important this was. Thankfully, Cherie and a number of dedicated professors aligned with her and supported her. Together, they changed the campus and how people learn. Matilda didn't get a chance to see this initiative all the way through since she went to graduate school somewhere else, yet I did.

My clients who never met Matilda told me how affirming it was for them to sit in chairs that suited them in their current body. As years passed and new students attended that university, they never knew a time without accessible seating. I think about all the freed-up space in their minds instead of being preoccupied with how to attend another lecture in pain. Matilda caused a ripple effect of freedom, and hundreds of people have already benefited from her advocacy.

Matilda and I met monthly as she started graduate school then moved our meetings to quarterly as she juggled her PhD. I usually cry at the end of my time with clients, and this meeting with Matilda I did, too. I like to do a sort of transitional activity at the end of all the meetings with clients if we can. Matilda chose to write a Love Food letter on her own. She wanted to sum up all the work she had done and keep it close. We both had tears rolling down our cheeks as she pulled out her phone's notes app to read her letter:

Dear Matilda,

For so long, you were told to cut out things to make yourself smaller. We love that you see that adding, not taking away, helps you stay awake to what needs to change and take up all the space you need. Thank you for helping others feel safer in the space they take up to remind them—and yourself—you don't need to be fixed. Next time you feel stuck or alone, remember, there's beauty in the differences and that's by design.

Love,
Food

Rae

Rae and I lost touch as they expanded their family. This happens sometimes as a dietitian. I am trained to leave my work at work yet sometimes people like Rae drift into my mind. Living in a small town, I run into clients often, but confidentiality—something I take seriously—keeps me from catching up. I saw Rae with their partner and children at an ice-cream shop. I heard laughter and saw messy ice-cream splats being wiped up with lots of napkins. I know life isn't always like a melting ice-cream cone, but I was grateful I got to see a glimpse of this.

After that sighting, I wrote down my own Love Food letter for Rae. Here it is:

Dear Rae,

You bring the world joy just by being in it. Stay connected to that. We wish the world had affirmed this all along, yet we are proud of the work you have done to rewrite your complicated food and body history. Your existence—with all its laughter, anger, and everything in between—makes the world better. Thank you for showing up and being you.

Love,
Food

Paul

Paul and I had our last session online. I felt funny sitting alone on the green couch as he told me about how he now defines his relationship with food. After working together for almost two years, he was ready to not set any further appointments. I knew he was ready, too.

"Tell that green couch you were right about one thing," Paul said. "I am not a food addict. I certainly felt like it and sometimes I still do. In those moments, I ground myself and can usually piece together something that is keeping me from eating enough."

I ended up working with Paul's spouse a few years later. As Gene and Paul decided on whether or not to have children, Gene wanted to work on her relationship with food, too. We met just a few times before they felt ready to move on. At our last session, Gene read me her note from Food:

> Dear Gene and Paul,
>
> Food had too much power and not enough at the same time within your lives. We see how shifting perspectives gave you insight into how to meet your own needs without another Diet Trap. Paul, we are glad you no longer hate us. Gene, we are rooting for you as you make these next steps wherever they go. Together, the two of you have all the insight into how to care for yourselves and your family. If you disconnect with that truth, remember to come back to the breath and the kitchen table. The flowers will remind you beauty is right in front of you.
>
> Love,
> Food

Elena

Elena is another person I lost touch with. Common with my busy teacher clients, our schedules started to not mesh well. We concluded our time together just as Elena was starting a new side project. After reconnecting with her favorite Mexican foods, she started bringing extras to share at the high school. People started to ask for her salsas in particular, and Elena loved making them. On a whim, she rented a booth at a small farmers' market. A few years after our work together ended, I heard my name while at my neighborhood's Saturday market. I turned around, and there was Elena handing me her salsas to try. Later that same night, Elena emailed me her Love, Food letter saying she wrote it on the way home:

Dear Elena,

The more you learn about yourself, the stronger you become. Always trust this. We know you overlooked or were trained to not acknowledge some parts, and we are glad you are holding on to every part of you. They are all important. We see how staying connected to your culture and its foods helps you bring your whole self to work. The students need all of you there, fed. Only then will these students make this a better world.

Love,
Food

Traci and Keisha

Traci emailed me to let me know a spot had opened up in a special travel-abroad opportunity at her university. This change meant we would not be able to meet the next month. We had been meeting monthly to give Traci a chance to vent about her pull back to scripts and ways to stay connected to her Food Voice. Her mom and I knew she was ready for this next step in independence, and from what I heard, studying abroad suited her. I lost touch with Traci yet got a card from her mom, Keisha, five years later. It included a graduation announcement—Traci had finished a graduate program in mental health counseling! Keisha tucked in a note: her letter from Food.

Dear Keisha and Traci,

The diet industry messed with the wrong family. You united to teach anyone who would listen how important eating enough was for the world. You stopped that school's weight-loss curriculum and got them to start a garden project instead. We see how Traci

231

quietly focused on fueling herself while also letting the world know she would no longer be quiet about injustices around her. We are so proud of you, Traci—helping kids recover from eating disorders. We see how your recovery has helped your mom to keep recovering, too. Remember, the world benefits from when you show up as you—even when your voice shakes.

Love,
Food

Dear Food letter activity

Dear Voice Finder,
   Are you ready to write your own letter from Food? Looking back at all the time and effort you have put into finding your Food Voice so far, what do you want to take with you? What do you want to let fall by the wayside? What encouragement do you need? Take your time and jot it down. Capture this meaning to provide the mirror reminding you how the world needs *you* fueled. We need you as *you*. Remember, there is nothing broken within you. You don't need to be fixed, but this world does. We hope you rally with us for the work ahead.

Love,
Food

Glossary

Check-In Props (CHIPs)   A time-based tool to help you practice noticing the present state of your mind, body, and soul. Scheduled about every two to three hours, CHIPs give you a speedbump during your busy day or downtime to consider your unmet needs. They help you connect with enough food and other means to sustain yourself as a human being. They are never meant to keep you from eating for any reason.

Curious Nutrition   A process of collecting data on adding new foods, movement, or rest to consider how these may impact your past, present, and future self. It relies on compassionate curiosity to explore new options in self-care. There is no good or bad outcome, and the person engaging in the process tries to detach themselves from the outcome without feelings of urgency.

diet industry   A $75 billion industry and economic activity serving 45-plus million Americans, including meal replacements, health clubs, weight-loss medications, supplements, diet drinks, technology companies, and anything related to making you look and eat a particular way.

diet trauma   The lasting physical, cognitive, and emotional reaction from unreliable access to food. Diet trauma can be caused by poverty, famine, neglect, or pressure to eat less.

Diet Trap   Through a predictable set of cultural desires, oppressive systems promise controlling food intake will lead to permanent weight loss, improved health, and increased safety and access. Because diets don't work for most people, the diet ends leading to weight cycling and self-blame for the diet not working. The desire for acceptance, access, and safety push the dieter to try again, resetting the cycle to continue.

emotional hunger   Yearning to eat without physical sensations. Just as with physical hunger, one has permission to eat with this cue.

food preoccupation   A predictable response in a human who is not eating enough, which provokes the brain to prioritize food thoughts over everything else. Sometimes referred to as *food addiction* or *food noise*, this is an evolved trait signaling the body's connection with receiving enough of a basic human need. Many people will describe feeling "out of control" or binge eating in response to food preoccupation. It is worsened with famine, neglect, restriction, dieting, or the threat of any of these. Also cued from diet trauma history.

Food Voice   An internal system each human is born with to communicate when to eat, how much, and what choices to consume based on what is available. This communication may be through body awareness like hunger, fullness, fatigue, mood, or satisfaction. This communication may also be through thoughts and feelings or guided by structured self-care techniques.

One's Food Voice will be unique to the individual yet always flexible, kind, and nurturing. Its primary function is to help the person prioritize eating enough. It is a knowing with unconditional permission for food yet compassionate when outside circumstances block access.

guardrails   Helping one access non-diet ways of eating while moving away from *I-Should-Eat* scripts, these tools include preselected check-in times and a series of questions used to help reconnect the mind, body, and soul. This redirects the mind to momentarily shift direction away from scripts and instead have a glimpse of one's kind, flexible, and nurturing Food Voice. Voice Finders have unlimited access to guardrails, and relying on them is not a failure. Some will need them only temporarily whereas others will need them for the rest of their lives.

***I-Should-Eat* script**   A seductive fantasy about eating less to earn power, access, and freedom, created by the diet industry and rooted in white supremacy. It tricks us into believing weight loss will happen after following a certain set of changing rules, but which in reality only keep us in the Diet Trap. It overpromises regarding the simplicity of weight loss and under-delivers on its guarantee for lasting thinness and all that comes from it. Everyone gets seduced by *I-Should-Eat* scripts in their lifetime. When one gets introduced depends on factors including how close you are to being thin, white, and cisgender, how much power you have in the world, and whether you are susceptible to an eating disorder.

intuitive eating   Created by Evelyn Tribole and Elyse Resch, a non-diet and self-care framework that combines physical, emotional, and logical experienes. It is weight inclusive and evidence-based with over 100 studies supporting its use.

meal hunger   Hunger has different degrees of intensity, and meal hunger has more depth, intensity, and need compared to snack hunger. Many report increasing borborygmi (intestinal noise), emptiness, and physical weakness with meal hunger. More food is required to provide satisfaction and fullness with meal hunger compared to snack hunger.

Nest Time   A protected space to create thoughts, visuals, or other connections to the healing work a Voice Finder needs. Typically needed daily, an individual sets aside protected time for safety (as much as this is possible), rest, or to gain support in community. It helps the Voice Finder stay connected, heal from past and present diet trauma, and navigate steps away from their Diet Trap.

non-diet honeymoon   Typically a temporary response when the drastic side of chronic diets meets raw permission to eat. It will feel as though the long-yearned-for blissful moments with food have finally come. The brain will feel a buzz as it finally has a break from constant food negativity.

panic hunger   Often described as an "out of control" eating experience, panic hunger is a deep required need to eat. It is normal when one's body doesn't get enough food and/or rest; it is sometimes predictable. When one experiences panic hunger, permission to eat will promote blood sugar stability, mood regulation, and healing. Everyone needs plenty of ready-to-eat shelf-stable foods that are enjoyable and feel energizing to create self-care in response to panic hunger.

physical hunger   Yearning to eat because of bodily alarms including stomach growling, noises, or emptiness; cognitive changes including food preoccupation and brain fog; and mood shifts including irritability and frustration (often referred to as being *hangry*).

snack hunger   Hunger has different degrees of intensity, and snack hunger has less depth, intensity, and need compared to meal hunger. Many report slight emptiness and distracting food thoughts with this type of hunger. It can be predictable or not.

Voice Finder   Someone unraveling their complicated history with food to understand how their body knows when, how, and what to eat without relying on the rules learned within oppressive systems or passed down through intergenerational food trauma. Voice Finders are healing and have permission to define their Food Voice in any way they choose.

weight cycling   A diet risk factor known to cause harm issues including higher mortality, higher risk of osteoporotic fractures, gallstone attacks, loss of muscle tissue, higher blood sugar, higher insulin levels, high blood pressure, chronic inflammation, and some forms of cancer. Repeated diet attempts, also called yoyo dieting, cause weight loss then regain. Most people who diet will weight cycle. It's important to note that dieting causes weight cycling and poorer health outcomes, not the dieter.

Resources

Books

Baker, J. (2018). *Landwhale: On Turning Insults into Nicknames, Why Body Image Is Hard, and How Diets Can Kiss My Ass.* Seal Press.

Burns, L. (2021). *Big & Bold: Yoga for the Plus-Size Woman.* Human Kinetics.

Gay, R. (2017). *Hunger: A Memoir of (My) Body.* HarperCollins.

Harrison, C. (2021). *ANTI-DIET: Reclaim Your Time, Money, Well-Being, and Happiness Through Intuitive Eating.* Little Brown Spark.

Harrison, D. (2021). *Belly of the Beast: The Politics of Anti-fatness as Anti-blackness.* North Atlantic Books.

Kater, K. J. (2005). *Healthy Body Image: Teaching kids to eat and love their bodies too!: promoting healthy body image, eating, fitness, nutrition and weight: a comprehensive resource manual and lesson guide with scripted-lessons and activities for grades four, five or six.* Eating Disorders Awareness And Prevention, Inc.

Kinsey, D. (2022). *Decolonizing Wellness.* BenBella Books.

Mann, T. (2017). *Secrets from the Eating Lab: The Science of Weight Loss, the Myth of Willpower, and Why You Should Never Diet Again.* Harper Wave.

Pershing, A., & Turner, C. (2018). *Binge Eating Disorder: The journey to recovery and beyond.* Routledge.

Strings, S. (2019). *Fearing the Black Body: The Racial Origins of Fat Phobia.* New York University Press.

Taylor, S. R. (2018). *The Body Is Not an Apology: The Power of Radical Self-Love.* Berrett-Koehler Publishers, Inc.

Tribole, E., & Resch, E. (2020). *Intuitive Eating: A Revolutionary Program That Works.* St. Martin's Essentials.

Walker, S. (2018). *Dietland.* Atlantic Books.

West, L. (2017). *Shrill.* Hachette Books.

Wilson, J. (2023). *It's Always Been Ours.* Hay House, Inc.

Podcasts

Burnt Toast with Virginia Sole-Smith

Diabetes Digital Podcast by Food Heaven with Wendy Lopez and Jessica Jones

Embodiment for the Rest of Us with Chavonne A. McClay and Jenn Jackson

Intuitive Eating for the Culture with Christyna Johnson

Maintenance Phase with Aubrey Gordon and Michael Hobbes

The Train Happy Podcast with Tally Rye

Appendix
Food Idea List

Use this list as you explore foods to add to your Curious Nutrition experiments. This list is in no way inclusive to all foods. If you don't see a food you want to try on this list, please try it! I appreciate foods come in different varieties, price points, and serving sizes so please keep in mind:

- Choose frozen, fresh, canned, pickled or however you enjoy the food and have access to it at the moment. No version is superior to another.
- The portion size is up to you and how much you have access to at the moment.

Adding carbohydrates

Potatoes (any kind)
Corn
Rice (white or any preferred variety)
Pasta
Tortillas
Bread (any variety)
Quinoa
Oats (instant, rolled, or stone ground)
Fufu
Barley
Farro
Rye
Couscous
Challah
Injera
Pizza
Millet
Beans
Lentils
Chickpeas
Hummus
Plantains
Yams or sweet potatoes
Taro
Bulgur
Polenta or grits
Orzo
Soba or rice noodles
Ready to eat cereal (sweetened or unsweetened)

Adding protein

Chicken
Turkey
Fish
Eggs
Duck
Yogurt (all types)
Green peas
Cottage cheese
Venison
Bison
Other game meat
Beef
Pork
Soy and soy milk
Shrimp
Lentils
Chickpeas

Seitan
Nutritional yeast
String cheese
Quinoa
Tofu
Tempeh
Edamame
Beans
Peanuts and peanut butter
Nuts and nut butters
Chia seeds
Milk
Cheese
Hemp seeds
Pumpkin seeds
Buckwheat

Adding fat

Butter
Peanut, canola, coconut, vegetable
    and all other oils
Fatback, lard, or schmaltz
Ghee
Full fat dairy
Avocado
Mayonnaise

Coconut milk
Olives
Cream cheese
Salad dressings
Nuts
Seeds
Chocolate (all varieties)
Egg yolks

Adding fruits

Apple
Banana
Orange
Strawberries
Grapes

Blueberries
Blackberries
Raspberries
Mango
Figs

Dates
Pineapple
Kiwi
Persimmon
Grapefruit
Apricots
Melon
Coconut
Nectarines

Peach
Pomegranate
Cherries
Pear
Plum
Papaya
Avocado
Lemon
Lime

Adding vegetables

Carrots
Broccoli
Peas
Spinach
Okra
Tomatoes
Peppers
Collards
Corn
Bok choy
Mustard greens
Potatoes
Cucumbers
Zucchini
Cauliflower
Pumpkin
Squash (butternut, spaghetti
    squash, or other variety)
Zucchini

Brussels sprouts
Green beans
Eggplant
Sweet potatoes
Cabbage
Celery
Swiss chard
Artichoke
Leek
Fennel
Kale
Beets
Asparagus
Lettuce
Radishes
Onions
Garlic
Mushrooms

Adding sweet tasting foods

Cookies (homemade or store
    bought)
Cupcakes

Ice cream or frozen yogurt
Chocolate
Macarons

Donuts

Pie

Candy

Gelato

Pudding

Pavlovas

Baklava

Trifles

Cheesecake

Crepes

Brownie

Eclairs

Mochi

S'mores

Churros

Popsicle

Adding salty or savory foods

Pretzels

Beef jerky or cured meats

Popcorn

Crackers

Potato chips

Onion rings

Nachos

Seaweed snacks

Tater tots

Salted edamame

French fries

Bagel chips

Cheese puffs

Tortilla chips

Salted nuts

Tostadas

Pickles

Salted chocolate

Olives

Pita chips

Takis

Adding fluids

Water

Vegetable juice

Coconut water

Smoothie

Sparkling water

Kefir

Fruit juice

Soup broth

Coffee

Ice tea (sweetened or

Soda

unsweetened)

Herbal tea

Lemonade

Milk

Kombucha

Sports drinks

Index

Notes